YOU CAN PREVENT A STROKE

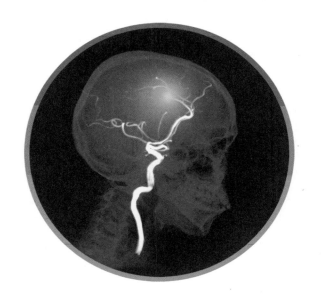

BY JOSHUA S. YAMAMOTO, M.D. F.A.C.C.
KRISTIN E. THOMAS, M.D.

The Foxhall Foundation

RosettaBooks®
NEW YORK, 2019

You Can Prevent a Stroke

Copyright © 2019 by Joshua S. Yamamoto and Kristin Thomas

First edition published 2019 by RosettaBooks
All photographs come from the personal archive of the authors unless credited otherwise.

Cover and interior design by Alexia Garaventa

ISBN-13 (print): 978-1-9481-2240-5
ISBN-13 (ebook): 978-0-7953-5225-6

Library of Congress Cataloging-in-Publication Data
Names: Yamamoto, Joshua S., author. | Thomas, Kristin.
Title: You can prevent a stroke / Joshua S. Yamamoto, M.D. F.A.C.C., Kristin Thomas, M.D.
Description: New York : RosettaBooks, 2019.
Identifiers: LCCN 2019011576 (print) | LCCN 2019012923 (ebook) ISBN 9780795352256 (ebook) | ISBN 9781948122405 (hardback)
Subjects: LCSH: Cerebrovascular disease--Prevention.
BISAC: MEDICAL / Cardiology. | MEDICAL / Preventive Medicine.
Classification: LCC RC388.5 (ebook) | LCC RC388.5 .Y36 2019 (print) DDC 616.8/105--dc23

www.RosettaBooks.com
Printed in Canada

RosettaBooks®

This book is dedicated
to our family and our patients.
You are all invited to our
retirement party, in 20 years...

ANIMUS FORTITUDO SAPIENTIA

**Grant me the SPIRIT to change
the things that I can,**

**The COURAGE to endure
the things that I cannot,**

**And the WISDOM to know
the difference.**

We are all destined to age. The process is no longer as mysterious as it once was. Some things are inevitable and must be endured, but the brain lives and dies by circulation. There is much we can do to keep our circulation healthy. There is much we can do to make sure our brain is not damaged from poor circulation. There is much we can do to prevent brain damage in ourselves and our loved ones. We can prevent strokes. We can prevent vascular dementia.

But only if we choose to.

THE FOXHALL FOUNDATION

The Foxhall Foundation is a not-for-profit organization dedicated to helping everyone age well. It was started in 2015 to help families take care of patients with dementia in the Washington, DC, area. It became evident that as we age, so much of dementia is a result of the brain damage related to strokes. So much of this damage was readily avoidable, and indeed preventable, but neither the general population nor their physicians had thought of strokes as being something that could, and should, be actively prevented.

After its inception, the Foundation began a program on stroke prevention. Foundation members give dozens of lectures and presentations on stroke prevention throughout the year to physicians and the community. These efforts lead to this book, which represents a summation of conversations we have with patients and colleagues every day.

All proceeds from the sales of this book go to support the Foundation.

FOR MORE INFORMATION, GO TO:
www.FoxhallFoundation.org

AUTHORS' NOTE

We, Dr. Thomas and Dr. Yamamoto, have been working together on and off since we were interns together at The Johns Hopkins Hospital in 1994. This book is really a compilation of the many discussions we have had with our patients over the years.

Contained within are many vignettes and encounters with patients. Although we may be married, we are not physically joined at the hips. Some encounters may have been with only one of us or the other, but we share a common thought process and routinely collaborate. In other words, throughout our text, we have written in the plural *we*. Mark Twain may have recommended that *We* be used only by Kings and people with lice, but perhaps he should have included close partners writing books as well.

That being said, occasionally Dr. Yamamoto will provide individual reflections and use the pronoun, *I*.

ABOUT THE AUTHORS

DR. THOMAS is a Michigan native who graduated with a degree in American history from the University of Michigan, and subsequently earned her medical degree there as well. She did her internship and residency on the Osler Medical Service at The Johns Hopkins Hospital. Upon completion of her training, she became the first "hospitalist" physician of Johns Hopkins before accepting the position of Assistant Chief of Service (Chief Resident). She gave up a promising academic career in the Department of Medicine at Johns Hopkins in order to marry a naval officer stationed at the National Naval Medical Center in Bethesda, Maryland. She then agreed to work with a prominent private medical practice in Washington, DC. Her husband joined her several years later when the two formed their own practice, Foxhall Medicine, PLLC. She has long been dedicated to the care of her patients and has watched them age, some more gracefully than others. In 2015, she started the Foxhall Foundation which initially worked to help provide services for patients with dementia.

DR. YAMAMOTO was born in Washington, DC. He graduated with a degree in physics from Princeton University, and subsequently worked as a paramedic for the Alexandria City Fire Department until he conned his way into Dartmouth Medical School. He too trained on the Osler Medical Service at The Johns Hopkins Hospital, and then completed cardiology training at the National Naval Medical Center and Georgetown University. He was the cardiology consultant to the US Congress and Director of Cardiac Imaging, and held a faculty appointment at the Uniformed Services University. In 2005, he was lent to the Army and served in Kuwait as the theater cardiologist for the ongoing wars in Iraq and Afghanistan. Upon his return, he dutifully followed orders and joined his wife in private practice.

TABLE OF CONTENTS

INTRODUCTION

I have been aggravated by many of my colleagues. The generation of physicians who preceded me were too often trained in the "old school." That is, if something isn't broken, don't fix it. A great emphasis was placed on symptoms. What are your complaints? If you don't have a complaint, then all must be well.

These same physicians accept that everything related to aging is inevitable. A famous bioethicist once said that there is no meaningful life after the age of 75, so why should anyone go to the doctor after that point?

In my practice, I can spend an entire day and see no patient younger than 90. And they are active and healthy, and enjoying life. I have 96-year-olds still wearing suits to the office. I have a 106-year-old complaining that no one will dance with her. I have an 89-year-old who wanted a stress test to make sure he could keep up with his new girlfriend (who in fact is older than he). I prescribe plenty of Viagra for a whole lot of people whom others would have written off because they are over 75. In fact, the census data now indicates that if you are 65 years old today, you can expect to live about another 20 years.

I am often also asked to see the spouses of many of my patients. Unfortunately, I often see them after a decade of neglect from their physician. They are old. They are slow. Their memory may be gone. They may have lost function of much of their body or suffered some other limitation from a stroke. And these aged spouses are often younger than my patients. How does it happen that my older patients are in better health than their younger spouses? There is no magic—just a little work and a lot of attention to detail.

I once tried to explain to one of my older colleagues how we practice cardiovascular medicine today. I tried to tell him that blood pressure is a number, not a disease. What matters is having good blood flow and not overworking the heart. I told him that we can measure how overworked a heart is with a simple ultrasound. I told him that the absence of chest pain does not mean someone is free from the risk of a heart attack or heart failure, but that you can look at a heart and watch someone exercise to know what their cardiac health is. I told him that if you want to know how healthy someone's arteries are, you can take five minutes and simply LOOK at the arteries with an ultrasound.

Explaining how the walls of arteries age, how the heart muscle ages, and how it is important to look at these things simply made this doctor's head spin. He finally threw up his hands in frustration and shouted, "You don't even care how someone FEELS, do you?"

I couldn't help but smile (inside) and try to console him. I responded, "I'm a cardiologist. I don't have that luxury. Symptoms do not predict risk."

I went on to say, "Using symptoms to look for heart and vascular disease is a lot like using an altimeter to look for a waterfall." When you are in a boat and it goes over a waterfall, you will drop rapidly. An altimeter will tell you that you are falling, but by then, this information is a little late to be useful. Often by the time you have symptoms, you have long missed an opportunity to make some simple changes that would have greatly affected your life.

Now, I consider myself a medical neo-libertarian. I feel that, as a physician, it is my job to give you my best advice. What you do with it is up to you. My colleagues may often aggravate me when they are out of date, passive, patronizing, overly basic, or simply lazy, but my patients rarely burden me. There are certain basic principles that apply to all of us, but every one of us is unique. Every one of us has our particular genetic fingerprint and our particular life experiences. We are allowed to have different bodies, different preferences, and different goals. That bioethicist who wants to quietly die at home at 75 is OK by me—as long as he doesn't drag his patients down with him.

Only once was I frustrated by a patient. He had chronic atrial fibrillation (an irregular heartbeat, which I will explain later). Suffice it to say, if you have atrial fibrillation, you have a high risk of stroke, unless you choose to prevent the stroke. The good news is that you can prevent strokes. But you have to believe a little of what your doctor tells you, and you have to take a pill.

A lot of people hate taking pills. I get that. I only prescribe them if it's for a good (and explainable) reason. This fellow was adamantly convinced that he had all of the answers. His condition was asymptomatic and therefore, apparently, didn't really exist. I always first try to reason with my patients. If that doesn't work, I charm them or cajole them. Before this man, I never resorted to bullying.

The problem was his wife was totally dependent on him. She had suffered a head injury years before and was absolutely dependent upon her husband for everything. They had no other family.

Try as I could, I was not able to convince this asymptomatic man that he still needed to take a pill to prevent having a stroke. Naturally, the call from the ER eventually came. I met him in his room, his wife at his side. By this point, the stroke had left him unable to speak. He was clearly dying. There was, however, still clarity in his eyes. He seemed to have a complete awareness that he was going to die. His eyes were angry.

I never was able to tell if he was angry that he was dying, angry that he had chosen wrong, or angry at seeing me. I was just angry that there was someone whose life depended on him who was now about to become a ward of the state. I was angry less at him and more at the situation.

I was angry because his stroke simply didn't have to happen.

It could have been prevented, but I failed to convince him of that.

So, if you don't want his fate, or the fate of his wife, read on.

Please.

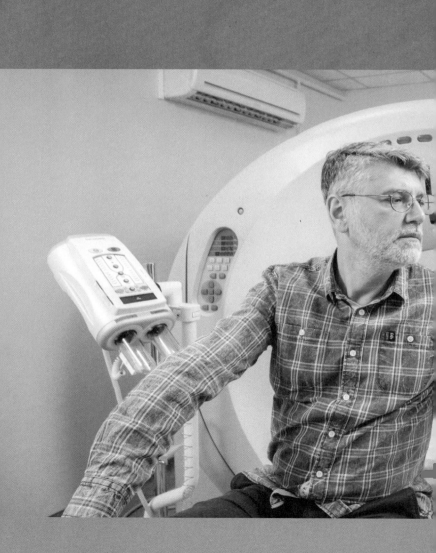

CHAPTER 1

"PREVENT" IS AN ACTIVE VERB

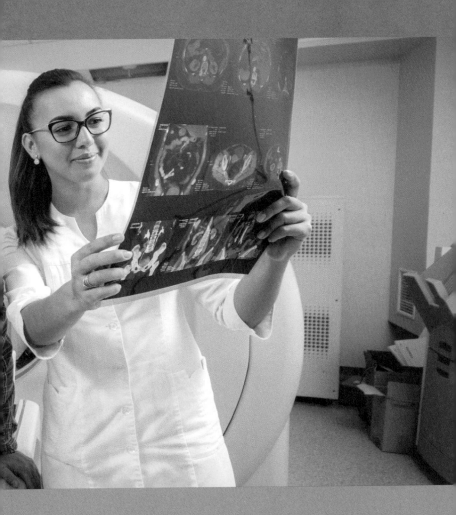

When I was in high school, I always liked to look in the back of the textbook to get the answers first. That way, I would know if I was on the right track in solving a problem. So, I will try to give the answers first.

To keep your brain (and yourself as a whole) healthy, know the answers to the questions:

1. What is the health of my heart and circulation?

2. What can I do, or what can I do differently, to keep my circulation working as SAFELY and EFFICIENTLY as possible?

Fundamentally, these are the only questions I ever get asked. The questions are simple, but the answers are different for all of us.

A few definitions are in order. First of all, what is a stroke? Technically speaking, we call a stroke a *cerebrovascular accident*. (As you can see, doctors love to confuse things by using Latin and Greek. I supposed lawyers are just as bad.) *Cerebro* means "brain." *Vascular* means "blood vessel," or refers to circulation. And accident, well, that always means something bad.

A stroke is damage to the brain caused by a problem with blood flow to the brain.
This is why cardiovascular doctors (also known as cardiologists) have always been responsible for *preventing* strokes, although they are not the doctors called when you *have* a stroke. The

doctors called when you have a stroke are neurologists (brain specialists). They should not be the first doctor you see to prevent a stroke. Hopefully, you will never need to see one. You should see your primary care doctor or a cardiologist first.

A stroke is not a heart attack. Sometime in the past 50 years, our medical vocabulary became even more confusing than it already was. The terms *stroke* and *heart attack* became interchangeable. They have a lot in common, but they are different things. A stroke is brain damage. A heart attack is heart damage.

Cardiologists prevent both. Historically we just have not been very aggressive about preventing strokes. Having a stroke means you have had brain damage, which means a neurologist (a brain specialist) will need to help you. Preventing a stroke means keeping your circulation healthy, which is not a job for a brain specialist. It's a job for a circulation specialist (that is, a cardiologist).

Biologically speaking, there are several types of strokes, but most of them are caused by a clot jamming up the blood flow to the brain. Those clots tend to come from the heart or the big blood vessels leading to the brain (the carotid arteries), or they can form in the smaller blood vessels within the brain. No matter what, you don't want blood clots in your brain. That's a stroke.

There are also "bleeding strokes," but they are not the common ones. In fact, many bleeds in the brain start as a clot. We tend to fear bleeding, but in fact, clots are a much, much bigger problem.

Clots can be prevented. That's part of how we prevent strokes.

A common question is what are the signs of a stroke? Well, the whole goal is to not have a stroke in the first place, but it is worth knowing what happens when you do clot off part of your brain. Remember, a stroke is brain damage. So, whatever part of the brain you damage may not work quite right again. It may not work at all. Pick a function that your brain controls. If you clot off the part of the brain that controls that function, it won't work. Just about anything related to brain function can be lost by a stroke.

For example, you may lose the ability to speak, to understand words, to see, to swallow, to move your arm or leg. You may not think right. You may be confused. Your face may droop. You may collapse. For better or worse, most strokes don't kill you. They just take something away, usually forever.

If you have a stroke, you will get to know a neurologist all too well. They are the experts who can tell you just how much of your brain has been damaged and how likely you are to recover what you have lost.

There are many books to help you understand how to recover from brain damage. This is not one of them. I find them all a little depressing.

If you do have a stroke, sometimes dramatic things can be done to try to rescue your brain. Several new studies have been published about some of these high-tech procedures (where tubes get stuck into your head to suck out clots, or clots are melted with drugs). One of my favorite patients recently asked me about these treatments. He wanted to know what was the best way to treat a stroke. The answer was really quite simple.

The best way to treat a stroke is to not have one in the first place.
What is a TIA? TIA stands for *transient ischemic attack*. They are often referred to as "ministrokes." *Transient* implies that you have symptoms that come and go. They are not permanent. *Ischemic* means some part of your body did not get enough blood. In this case, we are talking about part of the brain not getting blood. *Attack*, well, that's got to be bad.

A TIA is a transient ischemic attack, or ministroke, where symptoms spontaneously recover without permanent damage.
Having a TIA means that some part of your brain did not get enough blood, and it didn't work. Like with a stroke, any part of the brain may be at risk. The difference between a TIA

and a stroke is that a stroke leaves evidence of permanent damage.

Usually, that evidence of a TIA is seen with an MRI scan of your brain. If you have symptoms of some part of your brain not working, and the symptoms get better, and a brain scan shows no evidence of permanent damage (that is, a stroke), then consider yourself lucky. You have had a TIA. You have dodged a bullet. You need to think very hard about how you, and your doctor, are going to PREVENT your stroke, because it is coming.

You do not need to wait for symptoms before you actively prevent a stroke.

A scenario we see every day involves seemingly cryptic or mysterious terminology on a brain scan (MRI) report. Someone undergoes a brain MRI and there is evidence of an old stroke, or many old strokes. The MRI is read as "small vessel ischemic disease" or "age-related atrophy." All of this means that at some point, the brain did not get enough blood flow, blood flow was interrupted, or brain circulation clotted. It is entirely possible, and actually quite common, to find brain damage on MRI that you were never symptomatically aware of.

In the past, we often felt that these abnormal scans, in which the damage shown never presented symptomatically, were much like the proverbial tree falling in a forest. If no one is there to hear the tree fall, does it make a noise? If you never have any symptoms, does it matter that the MRI says you had a stroke?

If enough trees fall in the forest, there's no more forest. If enough of your brain gets damaged, you will eventually become demented.

OLD SCHOOL: In medical school, we learned to wait for someone to have a stroke before we did any investigation. The unfortunate patient would be admitted to the hospital under the care of the neurologists. They would meticulously examine the patient to determine what parts of the brain did not work, and correlate those findings with the brain scans (CT scans, and later MRI scans). We would order all sorts of tests to look at the heart and the blood vessels and monitor the heart rhythms to see if we could determine why someone had a stroke. The idea was, once we understood why your stroke happened, we just might do something to prevent the next one.

NEW SCHOOL: We know that strokes come from changes in how the heart and circulation work. We actually look for ways to prevent your first stroke, not your second, by knowing the health of your heart and arteries.

Vascular dementia is the loss of brain function, especially the ability to think, due to inadequate or interrupted blood flows.

There are actually several ways in which we can become demented. We tend to use terms like *Alzheimer's* and *dementia* interchangeably, but technically they are different. Dementia means that your brain doesn't work. Alzheimer's is a specific disease in which unusual proteins build up in the brain for unknown reasons. We have no good way of preventing or treating Alzheimer's. But some of what we think of as Alzheimer's is actually vascular dementia. And Mother Nature says you can have both. We may not be able to prevent Alzheimer's, but there is a lot that we can do to prevent vascular dementia.

We used to say that old folks simply became *senile*. The inference was that their memory was gone. Their ability to think rationally was gone. They were maybe a little goofy if not downright crazy. It finally evolved into an insult. If anyone was ever confused or forgetful, they were accused of being senile.

Well, technically, "senile" just means "old."

Natural aging predictably changes circulation. As circulation changes, blood flow to the brain can become less reliable. Clots form. Blood flow can be interrupted. The heart may not pump enough blood to the brain, and the brain suffers. Then you can in fact become "senile" if you develop vascular dementia.

Age is going to change circulation. It should come as no surprise that the brain suffers when circulation is inadequate.

Senility is vascular dementia. If you want to avoid it, keep the circulation to your brain healthy.

Perhaps the most important point is this: We do not need to simply accept growing old the way our grandparents did. We have the ability to keep the effects of time in check (at least when it comes to the heart and circulation). But we need to make the choice to be an active participant. We can prevent the changes to the heart and circulation that lead to strokes, brain damage, and vascular dementia. They do not prevent themselves.

The basics of prevention are already mentioned above: Know your heart and vascular health, and ask if you are doing everything you can to keep things working. Well, how does one do that?

What do we do to prevent strokes and vascular dementia?

- Establish a relationship with a physician.
- Know the health of your heart.

- Know the health of your arteries.

- Know the regularity of your heartbeat.

- Know if it's time to take a medicine to prevent plaque in your arteries and whether you need a pill to prevent a blood clot.

This is what we now call the **Foxhall Formula**, or protocol. It is a short list of steps everyone can take to make sure they are preventing strokes.

To prevent strokes, it may not take a whole village, but it does take a good relationship with a doctor. There are things you will need to do, and things you will need your doctor to do with you.

Notice the list does not mention diet or exercise. Of course fitness helps everything. A rational diet is important (more on that later), but if a magic fruit existed to keep our arteries perfectly clean and plaque free, I'd like to think we would have found it by now.

The list does include a lot of questions to be answered; fortunately they are all easy to answer—but you have to ask.

THE FOXHALL FORMULA

Steps to take to prevent a stroke; also called the **D-HART** strategy

D
DOCTOR
Have a doctor, and ask about your HART.

V2

V3

R

H
HEART
What's the health of my heart?

A
ARTERIES
What's the health of my arteries?

R
RHYTHM
Is my heart beating regularly and fast enough?

T
TIME
Is it time for a pill?

D First, establish a relationship with a physician. (D for Doctor)

The internet and "Dr. Google" are a great way to get information, but a dedicated physician is invaluable to help you navigate your health needs over the passage of time.

I ask all of my patients to see me at least once a year. Quite simply, even if you don't change in a year, sometimes we (doctors and health care providers) get smarter. You see, it is important to know all about your health, but knowing about your health is just the first step. The next step is working with your doctor to stay as healthy as possible.

H Know the health of your heart. (H for Heart)

When I trained at The Johns Hopkins Hospital, we had a saying: "The definition of a healthy person is someone who hasn't been fully evaluated yet." Asking questions is easy. It's what we do with the information that matters.

We call heart and vascular disease the "silent killer," because it does not always produce symptoms. It may be silent, but it is not invisible. We can see it, but first we have to look.

If you want to know your heart's health (which you do), then look. This is done easily with an echocardiogram (echo), which is an ultrasound of the heart. It's the same machine we use to look at babies in the womb. Painless, quick, harmless, non-invasive, cheap (and covered by Medicare for a whole lot of reasons), an echo will tell us about the strength of your heart, whether it's been damaged, whether it's been overworked by high blood pressure, whether your heart valves are healthy, and how much you are at risk for the irregular heartbeats that cause so many strokes.

An echocardiogram is really just part of the physical exam. There should be no guessing as to your heart's health when all you need to do is look.

CT scans (also called CAT scans) are great tools for many things, but they produce still images, and ultimately, the heart is a moving organ. Ultrasound (echo) allows you to see how a heart works because you can watch it move in real time. Resist the temptation to have a scan that gives you a still picture of your heart as your only test of heart function.

An echo is essential, but by itself it will tell you only how your heart works when you are sitting still. It is essential to know how your heart works when you are working. This is simple enough— have your doctor perform some form of stress test, preferably with exercise. That is, have your doctor watch your heart as you work. No one beats a treadmill. It can always go faster. Everyone will reach a limit. If your doctor watches you walk on a treadmill and takes pictures of your heart at the same time (a stress echocardiogram), it really does answer the question, what is the health of my heart?

Knowing the health of your heart is important. If your heart isn't healthy, you may not get blood to your brain, and your brain will suffer. Indeed, if your heart isn't healthy, that's just bad for everything.

 Know the health of your arteries. (A for Arteries)

The carotid arteries are the blood vessels in your neck that bring blood to your brain.

Knowing the health of your carotids is easy, and important. If your carotid arteries are full of gunk (also known as plaque), the gunk (and blood clots) can break off and get into your brain. A stroke.

If you want to know the health of your arteries (which you do), then look at them, again with an ultrasound. A high-resolution carotid ultrasound can be an invaluable tool to know the health of your arteries and guide your plan to prevent strokes.

R — Know the regularity of your heartbeat. (R for Rhythm)

As we age, the heart naturally tends to become slower and irregular.

Atrial fibrillation, or AFib, is what we call it when the heart beats in an irregular pattern. It is extremely common as we age, it is often asymptomatic, and it is a major cause of strokes that can be prevented.

If your heart is beating irregularly, you may not know it, but it matters. You may benefit from some form of cardiac monitor, especially a long-term cardiac monitor, to know for sure whether or not you are having an irregular heartbeat.

Also, if your heart is too slow, it may simply not be pumping enough blood to your brain. A chronically slow heart is one of the most preventable but under-recognized causes of dementia. A pacemaker may be a solution. Much more on irregular heartbeats, AFib, and pacemakers later.

T — Is it time for a pill? (T for Time)

We live in the 21st century. If we want to live the "all-natural" life, we must accept the fate of our ancestors who did not have modern medicine. Personal choices and lifestyle matter, but all the diet and exercise in the world will not change our genetics or make us exempt from the wear and tear of time. Once we do everything we can to lower our risks, what we are left with are the things we cannot change on our own. This is when your doctor can be helpful—determining what medicine in what dose at what time makes sense for you.

Statins are a family of medicines you might know by their trade names: Crestor (rosuvastatin), Lipitor (atorvastatin), Livalo (pitavastatin), Zocor (simvastatin), Pravachol (pravastatin), Mevacor (lovastatin), Lescol (fluvastatin). They work by keeping your arteries healthy, and they prevent strokes (more on that later too).

Most of us will benefit from statin therapy eventually.
Notice I did not say we need to treat cholesterol (although that helps). I said we have medicines that can keep our arteries healthy and prevent strokes and brain damage (and prevent heart attacks too!). In the past, we thought of the statins as medicines to treat cholesterol. Although they do lower cholesterol, they do much more.

We also have to ask what we are doing to prevent clots from forming too easily. Many people simply take a baby aspirin, which is often very helpful. Some people can't or shouldn't take aspirin. A lot of people need a direct oral anticoagulant (DOAC) like Xarelto or Eliquis. Anticoagulants prevent clots.

TOO MUCH OR TOO LITTLE?

Two studies came out back-to-back in the fall of 2018. One said that we aren't taking enough aspirin to prevent strokes, and the other said that we didn't need to take aspirin at all. What are we to believe? If you look at the details, in the first study, patients had more plaque in their arteries, or more advanced aging of their hearts and blood vessels. In the second study, almost everyone had been working with their doctors to aggressively prevent vascular aging by taking multiple mediations. In that study, anyone with plaque in their arteries was excluded.

The point is, treatment is not one size fits all. Some of us need very aggressive medication to prevent clotting, and some do not need much of anything. The more we prevent clotting, the more we encourage bleeding. A doctor can help sort this out.

Most of us eventually need something to prevent clotting if we want to prevent strokes.

Of course, the more we prevent clotting, the more we encourage bleeding. This may be one of the hardest things to accept. We tend to naturally want to avoid things that make us bleed, but we have to face the reality that most brain damage comes from clotting.

Choosing to do nothing is still a choice. We must all ask, what am I doing to prevent a stroke?

NOTES:

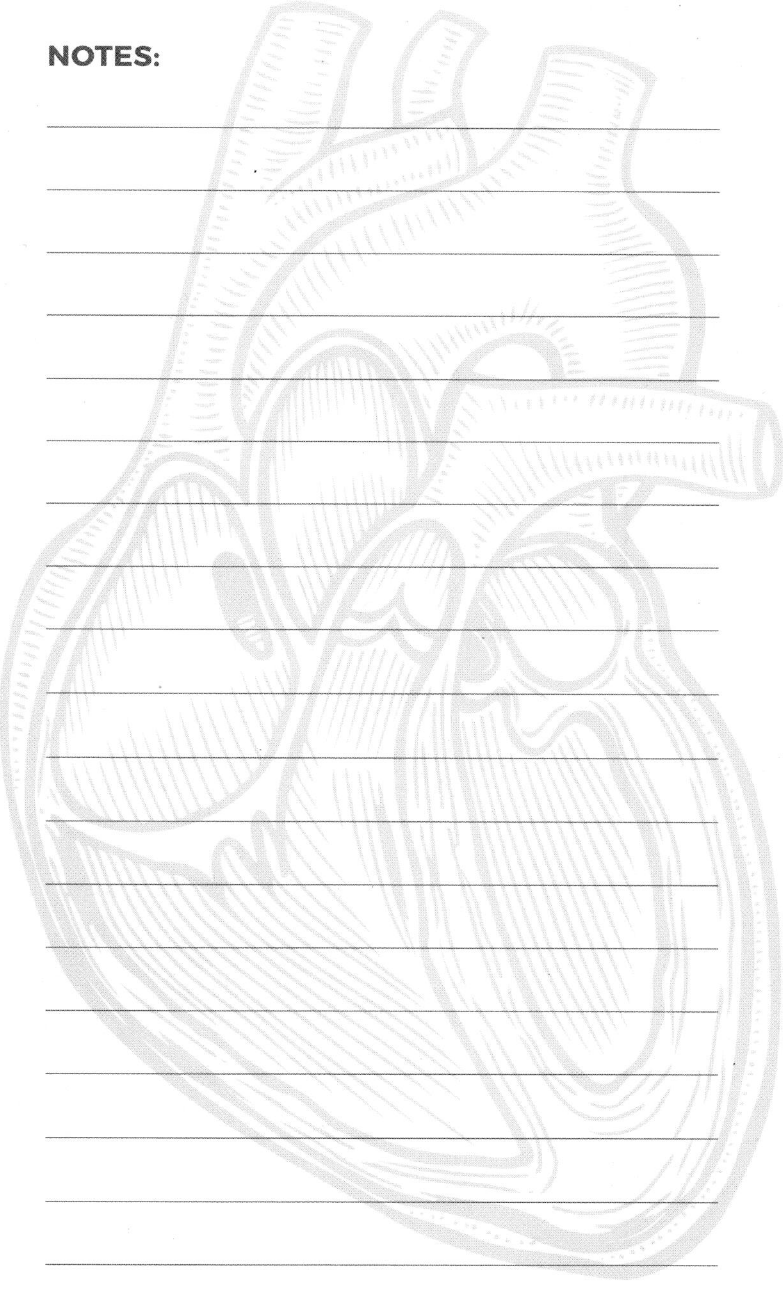

_____

_____

_____

_____

_____

_____

_____

_____

_____

_____

_____

_____

_____

_____

_____

_____

_____

_____

_____

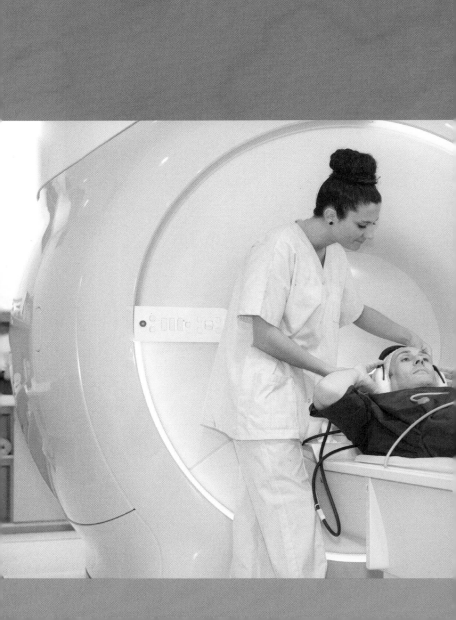

CHAPTER 2

DO YOU REALLY THINK YOU ARE IMMUNE FROM TIME?

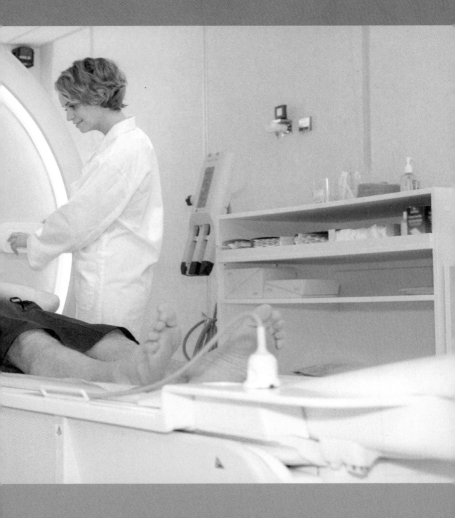

There are at least three notable things that will happen to our circulation over time simply because we age: chronic vascular inflammation, loss of vascular compliance (or "stretchiness"), and a decline in our heart's tempo.

One hundred thousand years ago, humans died of wounds, infections, bleeding, and malnutrition. Ancient cave dwellers did not live long enough to get any of our 21st-century diseases, like heart attacks, strokes, lung cancer, colon cancer, and breast cancer (the current leading causes of death).

In order to survive, we had to be good at healing so we would not die of our injuries. We had to be good at fighting infections. We had to be good at clotting, or we bled to death. We had to store calories well. Survival of the fittest, as Darwin would say, means that we have genetically selected ourselves to heal and clot well.

The body's healing mechanism is known as inflammation. We use the term *immunity* when we talk about our ability to fight infection. We use the term *inflammation* when we talk about repairing injury. They are all part of the same system.

Our genetics determine how robust our inflammatory system is. We are genetically programmed to heal injuries. Those who heal the best win.

That's all well and good, if you are young and wrestling sabretooth tigers, but after a few decades of life, all the healing can leave its mark. Quite literally, healing is what gives us scars. Now, imagine how that affects the *inside* of our bodies.

We have 100,000 heartbeats a day. That's a lot of wear and tear.

Snap your fingers a few times. How did that feel? Not too bad. Now do it 100 times. How about 1000 times? How about once a second for 24 hours? How about doing that all year? How about 65 years? You would tear the skin off your hands.

That is essentially what is happening inside our arteries every day. Our arteries are pipes carrying blood away from our heart to every part of our body. Arteries are made of living tissue. They have a lining of cells. This lining is constantly being pounded on by the pressure waves of blood coming from our hearts. That relentless pounding causes stretching and tearing on a microscopic level. The body, fortunately, heals this tearing. We are in a constant state of healing of our blood vessels. This is known as chronic vascular inflammation.

One of the key components of aging is chronic vascular inflammation.

Simply put, life itself is traumatic. A pumping

heart is a moving part. Pounding on our blood vessels causes damage that we are constantly healing. That healing mechanism in blood vessels results in what we call *atherosclerosis*, or plaque. It is kind of like forming a scab or a scar, only on the inside.

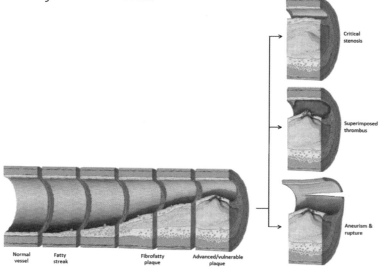

Critical
stenosis

Superimposed
thrombus

Aneurism &
rupture

Normal
vessel

Fatty
streak

Fibrofatty
plaque

Advanced/vulnerable
plaque

Atherosclerosis: the progressive process of growing plaque in an artery. It is the result of chronic inflammation, or the wear and tear of time on an artery.

Plaque in blood vessels, or atherosclerosis, is not a disease. It is a natural part of aging. Plaque is not something that sticks to an artery. Plaque *grows* in the walls of arteries. It is part of the natural healing process. It is not simply made of cholesterol. It is dynamic. It changes as it ages, progresses, and grows. It is a mix of healing blood cells (white blood cells), clot, fibrous bands, and the lipids (fat and cholesterol) that fuel inflammation. Eventually it stabilizes and hardens, a little like a growing coral reef.

This is one of the most important realizations of modern medicine. Our own healing process, inflammation, is what gives us plaque.

Everyone heals. If you can't heal, you don't survive. Circulation is traumatic. As we heal from the damage, we all grow plaque in our arteries.

Plaque in the arteries of our brain is a major cause of strokes and brain damage.
If you have enough plaque, it can block blood flow. If blood is blocked from flowing downstream, then whatever is waiting for that blood dies. If it was your brain that was waiting for blood, it dies. That's a stroke. If enough of the brain dies, you get vascular dementia.

But you do not have to completely block your artery with plaque to have a stroke. When plaque begins to grow, it acts a lot like rust in a pipe. A pipe, like an artery, should be smooth. As rust forms, the pipe becomes rough. Little pieces can break off and block flow downstream. Small blood clots can form in the nooks and crannies of plaque and then break free and travel down the arteries. They will eventually get stuck in the smaller branches of your arteries and completely block flow. Again, once flow is blocked, something starts to die.

A small blood clot that forms on plaque and breaks free, and then gets stuck downstream blocking blood flow in the brain, is a very common cause of strokes.
You do not want plaque, but it is going to happen. Unless, of course, you prevent it.

The more plaque you have, the more likely you are to have a stroke. Plaque is also the mechanism of heart attacks. The heart pumps blood to itself. It has its own blood supply that feeds oxygen to the heart muscle and electrical cells. A heart attack is when blood flow to the heart muscle is blocked by plaque and clot. When that happens, the heart muscle dies. When clot and plaque block the arteries in the brain, that's a stroke, and the brain dies. Brains have strokes. Hearts have heart attacks. They are a lot alike.

The main blood vessels bringing blood to the brain are the carotid arteries.
These are the big pipes of blood that give us a pulse in the neck, one on each side. Carotid arteries bring blood from the heart to the brain. The jugular veins reverse the route, returning blood from the brain to the heart.

They are right next to each other in the neck. (The veins are actually not all that important, although I never want anyone to "go for my jugular." An awful lot of blood goes into and out of our brains!)

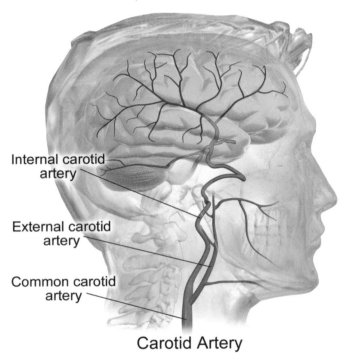

Carotid Artery

Carotid arteries bring blood from the heart to the brain.

How much plaque we have in our carotid arteries matters a lot. You do not have to block the artery to have a stroke. All you need is enough plaque to let a clot form, and have that clot break off and land in the brain. Then you will have a stroke.

When we look at a carotid artery with an ultrasound, we can see through the walls of the artery. We can see how much plaque you are growing. We call this your *plaque burden*. You can have a lot of plaque but no blockage.

Remember my favorite doctor (you know, the one more concerned about feelings than risk)? I once described to him the carotid arteries of a mutual patient. I told him that the patient had an extensive plaque burden in his carotid arteries, but no significant blockage. Once again, his head spun, and he was completely baffled. "How can you have extensive plaque without a blockage?" To this day, I suspect he thinks I'm off my rocker.

It's simple, really. If a pipe is lined with rust from one end to the other, it has extensive rust, even if that rust is not blocking flow through the pipe.

Your carotid arteries do not have to be blocked for you to be at risk of a stroke.
Remember: plaque forms naturally from the trauma of time. We clot naturally. That means time alone will give us plaque, clots, and strokes. So do we simply accept this? Of course not. (You wouldn't still be reading if we did.)

We can prevent plaque. We can prevent atherosclerosis.

First, the hard stuff. Plaque in our arteries may be a natural part of aging, but we don't have to encourage it. There are things that accelerate natural vascular aging. We used to call these *risk factors*. I think that the term is horribly outdated and deceptive. It is deceptive because it implies that if we eliminate all of the risk factors, you will never have vascular disease.

Well, it's not a disease. It's natural aging. I realize that I may be harping on this point, but it is very, very important: Atherosclerosis is not a disease. It is natural aging. We just don't want to speed it up.

The main things that accelerate natural vascular aging are:

- Diabetes

- Smoking

- High cholesterol (hyperlipidemia)

- High blood pressure (hypertension)

These are also commonly called *modifiable risk factors*. Simply put, we can actively choose to do things to control diabetes, smoking, blood pressure, and cholesterol.

OLD SCHOOL: All doctors are taught to help patients reduce the risk factors for heart disease. These risk factors include high cholesterol, high blood pressure, diabetes, and smoking. This is all important to do, but it is not the end of our effort to prevent strokes, heart attacks, dementia, and death.

NEW SCHOOL: We prevent plaque formation. We modify the things that accelerate vascular aging (see above) and then we decide how aggressively we need to act to prevent the growth of atherosclerotic plaque. We treat to prevent plaque growth, not just modify risk factors.

You cannot change your genetics, and you cannot change the fact that time passes. We can, however, cheat. (More on that later.)

Dealing with the things that accelerate vascular aging is the first and hardest thing we need to do. This takes a lot of effort.

Take smoking. Simple. Don't smoke. But if you've started, stopping isn't easy. Try anyway. Then try again. On average, it takes about seven attempts at stopping smoking before anyone is successful. I'm not here to tell you how to stop smoking. There are many, many other sources of help for that. I'm just here to tell you that smoking accelerates vascular aging. If you're lucky, you just have a big heart attack and die quickly. Otherwise, you will die slowly, suffering brain damage from strokes or any number of awful cancers. Too harsh? Like I said, simple to say, not easy to do.

Diabetes. Now that's really tough, but worth the effort. Diabetes accelerates vascular aging very quickly. It is at least as bad as smoking, if not worse. Adult onset diabetes, also called type 2 diabetes, is the metabolic condition where we no longer process sugar as well as we need to. Our bodies use sugar as energy for everything that we do. Much of what we eat gets broken down into sugar. If we don't burn that sugar, we store it. Our body produces insulin in order to burn that sugar.

Over time, many of us are genetically programmed to store calories. We can become resistant to insulin, and the sugar level in our blood runs higher than needed. If we are resistant enough to insulin and our sugar level is high enough, we call that diabetes.

Remember, our caveman ancestors had to guard against starvation, famine, and the coming Ice Age. Those who stored calories most efficiently won. But in the 21st century, we have calories in abundance, and we do not have to put much effort into getting them. It is entirely possible to get on your cell phone and have all the calories in the world delivered to you without burning any energy at all. Our ancestors genetically selected us to store calories so well that now we all need to be mindful of our risk of developing diabetes.

So, hypothetically, we are all either pre-diabetic or diabetic already.

We care about diabetes because it accelerates vascular aging.
Anyone with diabetes will have accelerated vascular aging, and has the potential to grow plaque in their arteries much more quickly than someone without diabetes. There is much we can do, especially in terms of our diet and exercise, that will directly improve our metabolism, prevent or manage our risk of diabetes, and thus improve our vascular health.

But all the dieting in the world will not prevent the effects of time on your circulation.
No matter how much diet may help (or not), time always passes. There is always some level of chronic vascular inflammation. You can never eliminate inflammation entirely. Preventing and treating diabetes is very challenging, but it does pay off. Diabetic control through diet,

exercise, and medications (if necessary) will prevent some acceleration of vascular aging.

Cholesterol and blood pressure are conceptually easier to handle than smoking cessation and diabetic control. Diet and exercise both play a role in the management of cholesterol and pressure, but ultimately, they can both be handled with pills if need be. What is important to note is that plaque in arteries is the end result of chronic vascular inflammation. It is not simply a matter of cholesterol control.

Your cholesterol numbers can be perfect and you will still eventually grow plaque.
Remember, the goal is to prevent stroke, brain damage, heart attack, and premature death. The goal is not to have nice numbers on your blood tests. The good news is that you can control many of the factors that accelerate vascular aging. The better news is that if you are willing to take a simple medication (a statin), you can directly inhibit vascular inflammation, and thus prevent most plaque growth. Statins cheat time.

Statin medications directly prevent vascular inflammation and plaque growth. They are vascular protective medications, not just cholesterol medications.
Chronic vascular inflammation is the first effect of aging that leads to strokes. The second

is a loss of vascular compliance. Simply put, our arteries stiffen with time.

Our arteries are made in large part of the protein collagen. Collagen changes over time. It becomes stiffer and loses its elasticity. It's the same reason our skin stiffens and wrinkles and our hair becomes brittle.

So, our arteries become stiffer over time.
Age gives us stiffer pipes. Stiffer pipes means higher pressure. Higher pressure means more work for the heart. More work for the heart means changes in how the heart functions. Many of these changes cause a lot of problems. These changes in our heart, if not well managed, will change our circulation and affect how well we can get blood to our brain. We will spend more time in the next few chapters on what this means and what we can do about it. A good diet and exercise program are helpful, but time alone will lead to stiffer arteries no matter what we do or what we eat.

Stiffer arteries are not the same thing as plaque in arteries. Both will naturally happen over time, but nothing says that both will happen in everyone at the same rate. That is, you can avoid plaque but still have stiff arteries, and vice-versa.

Thirdly, everyone's heart tends to slow down with time. Have you ever gone to the gym and looked at that chart on the wall that says what your target heart rate is for your age? The line has a steady downward slope. Just like everything else, the older we get, the less well things work.

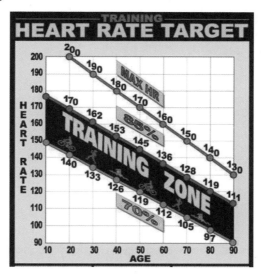

The ability for our heart to speed up will diminish over time. Basically, everyone's heart tends to get slower as we age. A slow heart when we are young is a sign of fitness. A slow heart when we are old basically means we are just old. A heart that is too slow will eventually be a problem.

Heart rate (or pulse) is the number of times our heart beats in a minute. Blood pressure is the force behind those heartbeats.

When it comes to heart rate, the slowing is predictable over time. In fact, there is a formula for it. Our maximum heart rate, on average, is

220 minus our age. That means a 20-year-old can get their heart beating 200 times a minute. An 80-year-old can get their heart beating only 140 times a minute (which in fact is quite fast).

That doesn't mean that an 80-year-old can't outrun a 20-year-old. I have an 85-year-old patient who is an avid runner and can outrace almost any 20-year-old I know. He just needed a pacemaker to do it.

Age does not mean you have to become unfit. The key point that I want to get across is this: You can do everything right, and time will still pass. You will still age. Some aspects of aging you can influence on your own. Some you cannot, at least not without your doctor's help.

There is (almost) no such thing as heart disease. It's mostly just natural aging. Natural aging leads to:

- Atherosclerosis (artery plaque) from chronic inflammation

- High blood pressure (from stiffening arteries)

- Slower and irregular heartbeats (like atrial fibrillation—much more on that later).

You are not immune from aging.

If all goes well, we age. Aging changes circulation. This change in circulation, if not managed well, leads to a failing heart, inadequate blood flow to the brain, strokes, vascular dementia, and senility.

One hundred thousand years ago, dying of old age meant that you survived childhood and child bearing, and died of an injury or starvation.

One hundred years ago, dying of old age meant that you died of pneumonia (an infection). "Pneumonia is an old man's friend" was the old expression.

Twenty years ago, dying of old age meant having a heart attack.

Today, dying of old age means senility, dementia, and heart failure.

Once again, we understand aging better than we did in the past. Aging is predictable, measurable, and manageable.

It has been said that the first person who is going to live to be 150 years old has already been born. I would not be at all surprised. I used to worry that all of my 80-year-old patients were going to die during my career. Now I know that most will not. So, if you're going to be alive, you may as well avoid heart failure and brain failure. If you are going to live, live well.

Remember the Foxhall Formula, D-HART

THE FOXHALL FORMULA

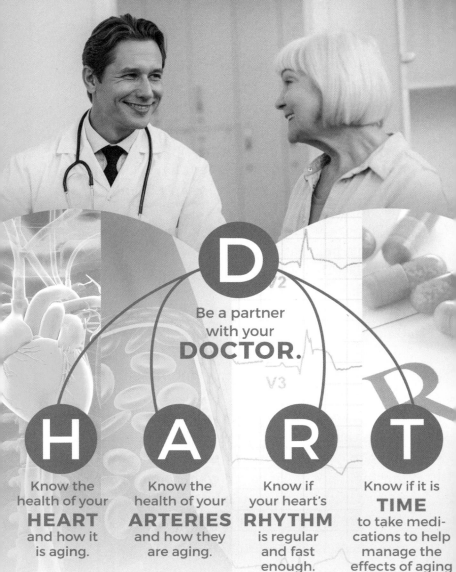

D
Be a partner with your **DOCTOR.**

H
Know the health of your **HEART** and how it is aging.

A
Know the health of your **ARTERIES** and how they are aging.

R
Know if your heart's **RHYTHM** is regular and fast enough.

T
Know if it is **TIME** to take medications to help manage the effects of aging that are not in your control.

AND, don't forget what part you can play in keeping yourself healthy as well.

NOTES:

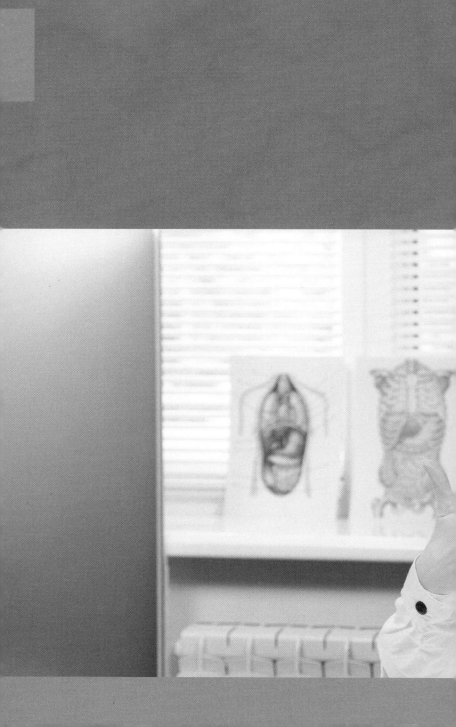

CHAPTER 3

ATRIAL FIBRILLATION (PART I):
IT'S COMING. DON'T TAKE IT PERSONALLY.

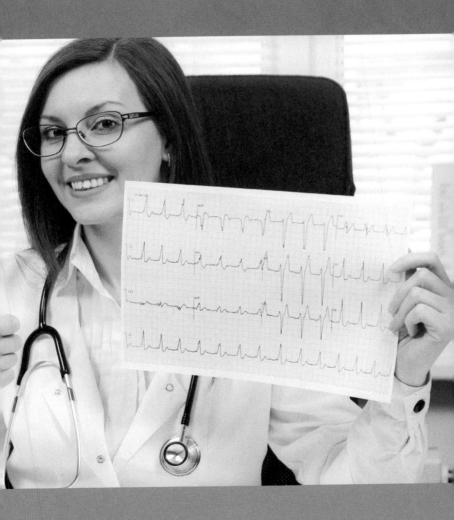

When my youngest son started third grade, I went to his classroom for Back to School Night. The students had all been asked to leave their parents a note with whatever message they thought was important. My son left me the shortest note in the class. It simply said, "Dad, pay attention."

That sage advice from a third-grader applies here. Atrial fibrillation, or AFib, is very important. It is very, very common, and it is possibly the most important factor driving strokes that can, and should, be prevented. I will explain what AFib is, why it is so very common, why it matters, and what you can do to prevent strokes.

Atrial fibrillation, or AFib, is very common, and it is a major reason why we have strokes. So, pay attention.

To understand AFib, it is helpful to spend a moment to understand how the heart normally works. The heart is a delightfully simple organ. It is just a pump. It is a hollow muscle that does nothing more than squeeze (or contract).

All of the blood in our body returns through veins to collect in the right side of the heart. The first chamber of the heart is the entry chamber, or right atrium. (The first room we enter in a church or large building is also called the atrium.) The atrium is at the top of the heart. Blood returns from the body to the top of the heart into the right atrium.

Blood leaves the right atrium through a valve into the next chamber, the right ventricle. Ventricles are the pumps. They are the lower chambers of the heart. Blood from the right atrium (the entry chamber) flows into the pump called the right ventricle. When the pump squeezes, blood is pumped out of the right ventricle through another valve into the lungs. This is usually an easy thing for the heart to do as the lungs are pretty darn close to the heart.

Blood passes through the lungs, picking up oxygen that we breathe in, and dropping off carbon dioxide that we breathe out. Blood then leaves the lungs and collects on the left side of the heart into the left-sided entry chamber, called (you guessed it) the left atrium. Blood leaves the left atrium through a valve called the mitral valve into the main pump of the heart, the left ventricle. The left ventricle is the largest, strongest part of the heart. When it squeezes (or contracts), it pumps blood throughout the entire body. Blood leaves the left ventricle through another valve, the aortic valve, to be carried by our arteries throughout the body.

The path of blood flow is this: Blood from the body goes through veins to the right heart.

From the right heart to the lungs. From the lungs to the left heart. From the left heart through arteries to the body (and brain!), and then back again.

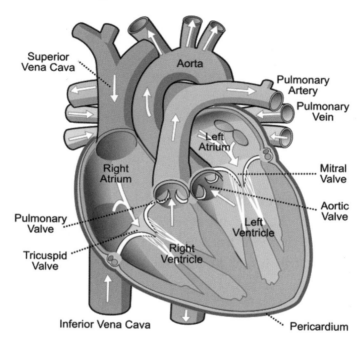

The anatomy of the heart. Blood returns from the body through veins into the right atrium, then enters the right ventricle, where it is pumped into the lungs. Blood returns from the lungs to the left atrium, passes into the left ventricle, and is then pumped to the body.

The atria (left and right) are the top, or upper, chambers of the heart. They are relatively passive and mostly collect blood to pass into the pumping chambers—the lower chambers, called ventricles. Normally, a heart beats in two stages, the "lub-dub" of the heart: first the upper chambers, then the lower chambers.

The heart, as mentioned, is just a muscle. It beats when it is told to beat. I like to compare the heart to a marching band. The band is supposed to keep in step. To stay in step, the band has a drum major who calls out the tempo. The heart has a natural drum major that spontaneously sends out a signal for the heart to beat. The heart's natural pacemaker is called the *sinus node*. A normal heart rhythm is called *sinus rhythm.*

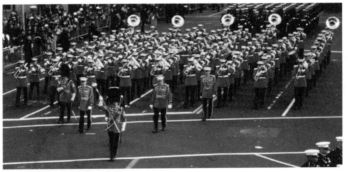

Normal Sinus Rhythm (NSR)

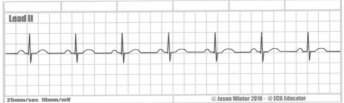

Lead II

25mm/sec 10mm/mV   © Jason Winter 2016 - @ ECG Educator

The heart marches to the tempo set by its natural pacemaker (the sinus node), just like a marching band keeps in step with its drum major.

The heart is a muscle that beats in rhythm, much like a marching band marches in step to a drum major.

Now, the heart is just a muscle, but it is a special muscle. My massive arm will flex only when my brain tells it to flex. My heart does not need my brain to tell it to beat. The heart has its own drum major telling it to beat. What's more, the heart really likes to beat. It likes to beat so much that any cell in the heart can try to start a heartbeat.

Every single heart muscle cell has a quality known as *automaticity*. That means that every single muscle cell of the heart can try to start its own heartbeat. If we think of our marching band, there is a single drum major that is calling the tempo for the band, but any member of the band can try to shout out to get the band to take an extra step.

The band, or the heart, often has someone calling out for extra steps. These are the occasional "skipped" heartbeats that everyone has. They are harmless as long as your heart is healthy and as long as your heart does not get entirely out of rhythm.

If your heart, like a marching band, completely ignores its drum major and gets entirely out of step, we call that atrial fibrillation.

Having been in a marching band in high school (couldn't you tell?), I can say with authority that any band, under the right circumstances, can get completely out of step. What's more, when the band doesn't have someone calling out a tempo, it easily runs out of control. The band members tend to run around chaotically without coordination or purpose.

The heart rhythm of atrial fibrillation has classically been called "irregularly irregular." We call this disorganized rhythm atrial fibrillation because when it occurs, the entry chambers of the heart (the atria) are so chaotic that they quiver. We call that quivering *fibrillation*. In AFib, the atria quiver without any useful contraction. The ventricles (the pumps) still contract, but they have no sense of timing.

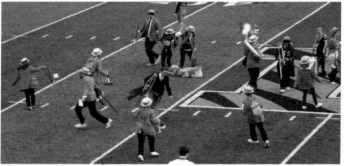

Atrial Fibrillation (AF)

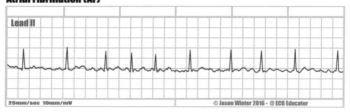

Lead II

25mm/sec 10mm/mV   © Jason Winter 2016 · @ ECG Educator

Atrial fibrillation is like the marching of a disorganized band.

Just because your heart is irregular does not mean that it is unhealthy.
The best musicians in the world can march in the most disorganized band in the world. There may be nothing wrong with the musicians at all, but if the band is not in step, it will still lack rhythm. Even a healthy heart can be in atrial fibrillation. In fact, in the right circumstance, absolutely any heart can be in atrial fibrillation. This does not have to be permanent, and, in fact, the heart often goes back and forth between atrial fibrillation and a normal rhythm. You may not even know it is happening.

There are many issues with AFib, but the most important issue is this: When the atria are fibrillating, they are not contracting well. They are just quivering. Without a good contraction, blood does not flow out of the atrium smoothly. The blood has a chance to pool inside the atrium. If blood pools long enough, it will start to clot. If a clot forms and leaves the heart, it tends to land in the brain, which is, of course, bad.

This is a very, very important point.

Atrial fibrillation is a MAJOR cause of strokes.
I promise there is good news. We can actually prevent these strokes almost entirely, but you are going to have to take a pill. Sorry, there's just no way around it. But first, more bad news.

Atrial fibrillation is very common. In fact, as I will explain, it really is a natural part of aging. It may be nearly universal if we live long enough. AFib is rare in anyone younger than the age of 50, but by the age of 80, nearly 40% of us will have AFib (if we bother to look). But, we don't always know we have AFib. In fact, nearly 90% of AFib is asymptomatic at first.

Want even scarier news? It takes only five minutes of AFib before you double your stroke risk.

Let's go over that again: AFib is common. Ninety percent of AFib does not produce symptoms. It is common to go back and forth between AFib and a normal rhythm. It takes only five minutes of AFib to double your stroke risk.

(Don't give up. There is good news. Those willing to take a pill can prevent those strokes!)

Now, remember my friend, "Dr. Feel-Good?" There is a very important but inconvenient truth about cardiovascular disease in general and atrial fibrillation in particular:

Symptoms do NOT predict risk.
Your risk of a stroke actually has nothing whatsoever to do with whether or not you feel bad from atrial fibrillation.

Atrial fibrillation is often asymptomatic, but it still puts you at risk for a stroke whether you feel it or not.

OLD SCHOOL: *Palpitations* is what we call the symptom of an irregular heartbeat. Many people, women in particular, will frequently have symptomatic, irregular heartbeats. If the women were not continuously in AFib, we disregarded the symptom. Basically, we told them to not worry and did nothing.

NEW SCHOOL: The symptoms are not what predict the risk. We need to know if you are having AFib, whether symptomatic or not, if we want to know how to help you prevent strokes. You don't know if you don't look.

So why is AFib so common? Consider how circulation ages. Arteries stiffen. There is vascular inflammation, and the natural pacemaker of the heart slows. All of these things are part of normal aging. (See the preceding chapter. You are not immune from aging).

When your arteries stiffen, that increases blood pressure. Stiffer pipes means higher pressure. Higher pressure means more work for the heart.

When a muscle works harder, it will get bulky. As we'll discuss later, a bulky heart is actually not a good thing. When the left ventricle is bulky, the left atrium has a hard time pushing blood into it. That makes the left atrium stretch. This is called atrial enlargement.

Left Ventricle Hypertrophy

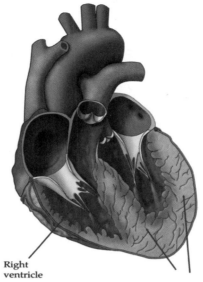

Right
ventricle

Hypertrophy

Overworked muscles can thicken. This may be desirable for body muscle, but if a heart muscle thickens, the heart will change shape. This leads to AFib. This is one reason why high blood pressure, which overworks and thickens the heart, leads to strokes. High blood pressure changes the heart and promotes AFib.

Increased atrial work and atrial stretch trigger the chronic inflammation that goes along with age. The atria will develop scar tissue (also called fibrosis). Atrial scar tissue is not as strong or flexible as healthy atrial tissue, and that makes the atria stretch even more.

A stretched, scarred atrium has a really hard time maintaining a regular electrical signal. Think of our marching band. When the band is spread out and beaten up, it has a hard time staying in step.

Age naturally leads to stiff arteries and high blood pressure. High blood pressure leads to increased work for the heart, which causes enlargement of the left atrium. Enlargement of the left atrium makes atrial fibrillation inevitable.

You see, it's really not your fault. Nor is it all in your control. In the four latest major studies on stroke prevention with AFib, of 60,000 people studied, nearly 90% had high blood pressure.

High blood pressure is a risk factor for strokes largely because it leads to AFib.

But wait. There's more. AFib is the rhythm of the heart when the heart is beating in a chaotic way. If we go back to our marching band analogy, we are in AFib when the band is out of step. When the band gets back in-step, we are back in a regular rhythm.

Every episode of AFib begins with a single, extra beat. There is always a first beat that starts the AFib. Imagine one guy in the back of the band who shouts at just the right time so everyone around him gets confused and no longer follows the drum major. The band will suddenly be out of step. Likewise, a single beat triggers every bout of AFib. These single beats are called premature atrial contractions (PACs) or atrial premature beats (APBs).

Atrial fibrillation is triggered by a PAC that originates in a stretched-out part of the left atrium (usually near or in the pulmonary veins). The more you have stretched out the atrium, the more likely you are to have PACs that can trigger AFib.

Remember how the heart muscle is special? It has what we call automaticity: Every single heart muscle cell is electrically active. Every single heart muscle cell can beat spontaneously. Heart muscle cells will beat when they are told to beat, but if no one tells them to beat, they will eventually beat on their own. This means we are all capable of irregularity. That's normal.

And it's a good thing.

Our heart really likes to beat. You would hate to think that if something happened to our drum major that the band would just stop. It doesn't. Somebody else in the band will try to call out the rhythm.

The heart will try relentlessly to beat, which is great. The price of this relentlessness is that all hearts can become irregular. All hearts can have AFib.

This is the part where the aging drum major comes in. The older the drum major is (that is, the older your heart is), the less reliable and slower it becomes. A slow heart encourages PACs. If the drum major doesn't call out a tempo, someone else in the band will. A PAC that comes from the right part of the atria will trigger AFib.

Age gives us stiffer pipes, which leads to higher pressure, which leads to an overworked heart, which leads to a stretched atrium. The natural pacemaker ages and slows, which encourages backup heartbeats (PACs). PACs in a stretched atrium trigger AFib.

The bottom line is this:

ATRIAL FIBRILLATION IS PART OF THE AGING PROCESS. IT MAY BE INEVITABLE IF WE LIVE LONG ENOUGH.

But that's ok. We can manage this.

As you might imagine, there is a lot that can be done to keep a heart healthy and fit so that you are less likely to have AFib. But don't feel too special (or cursed) if you do have AFib. Everyone can have AFib. It's how you manage it that matters. More on that shortly.

The formula is: *age + high blood pressure + a slow natural pacemaker = AFib.* You need to know the health of your heart (Has my atrium stretched?) and you need to know the health of your natural pacemaker.

Did I mention that AFib is a major cause of strokes? I'm sure I did. Don't want to have AFib?

Keep your heart healthy. Don't let high blood pressure beat up your heart. There's a reason our new blood pressure guidelines have us treating blood pressure more aggressively at an earlier age.

We will talk more later about what you can do to stay healthy, but did you ever wonder why exactly diet and exercise lower the risk of anything? For one, exercise keeps arteries from stiffening so much. This keeps blood pressure down, and decreases the work your heart has to do. When you decrease the work for your heart, you don't stretch out your atria, so you don't encourage AFib.

Like salt? Our bodies are mostly water. Actually, we are mostly saltwater. We are roughly a 1% salt solution, so for every gram of salt we eat, we have to hold on to 100 grams of water. The more water we have in our system, the more we pressurize those stiff pipes. That is, salt will increase our blood pressure, and—did you guess?—help stretch our atria and encourage AFib.

If you want to try to avoid AFib, treat your blood pressure early.
It is helpful to work with your doctor on treating blood pressure. Diet and exercise matter, but age and genetics play a strong role. Sometimes it's worth taking a pill.

So what causes AFib? Last I Googled that question, I got over 28 million results. "Cause" is really not the right question. All humans can have AFib. It's not some disease we catch like a virus. A better question is, what is my likelihood of having AFib? For that, just ask your doctor to look at your heart. Ask for an ultrasound of your heart (an echocardiogram, or *echo*). The ultrasound will tell your doctor just how well your blood pressure has been treated, whether your heart has been damaged, and whether your atria have been stretched out. An echo will tell your doctor an awful lot about how likely you are to have AFib.

If there really are 28 million web links about "causes of AFib," but *everyone* can actually have AFib, what are they all talking about? Many of them are talking about things that will damage a heart and increase the likelihood of AFib (like high blood pressure and arterial disease), and many of these sites are actually talking about "triggers" of AFib. Almost anything can trigger AFib. Probably at least 28 million things.

The first thing to remember is that AFib is a major cause of strokes, whether you know you have AFib or not.

But take heart. We can prevent strokes related to AFib. Read on.

NOTES:

_____

_____

_____

_____

_____

_____

_____

_____

_____

_____

_____

_____

_____

_____

_____

_____

_____

_____

_____

IT'S COMING. DON'T TAKE IT PERSONALLY.

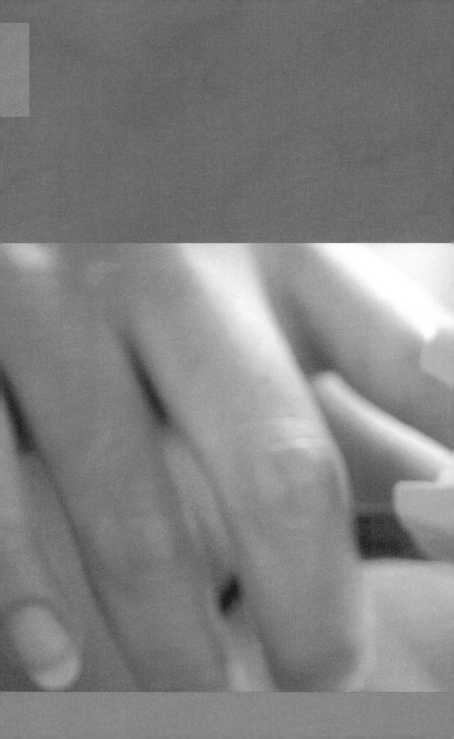

CHAPTER 4

ATRIAL FIBRILLATION (PART II):
SO YOU HAVE AFIB. DEAL WITH IT.

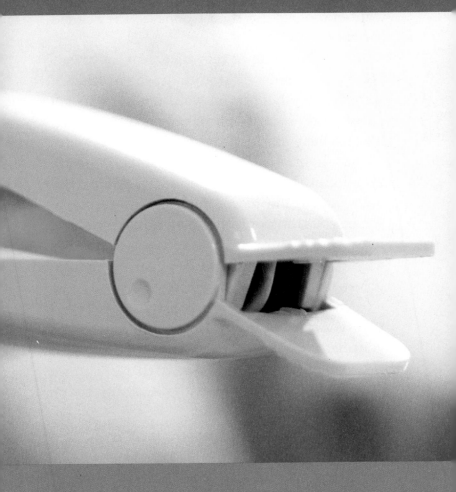

I used to serve as a Navy cardiologist. In 2004, the most common medical reason (not related to trauma) for the Army to send a soldier home was to see a cardiologist. We had tens of thousands of National Guardsmen deployed. Many of them were older. The Army finally realized that it would be easier to move one cardiologist than hundreds of soldiers. Naturally, the Army wanted the best for their troops, so they called the Navy.

I had the honor of serving a year in Kuwait, seeing hundreds of troops. It seems that if someone is shooting at you, it's easy to get chest pain (even if you have a healthy heart). It's also easy to go into AFib.

As I mentioned in the last chapter, there are 28 million things that can trigger AFib. They have something in common: stress response. When you think of it that way, it makes a little more sense. Our stress response is our body's way of dealing with danger. Anything that drives up stress can trigger AFib.

I gave our soldiers a simple message: I can't take your stress away. I can only make sure your heart can handle it.

We never completely cure AFib. Nor can we entirely prevent it. We just have to make sure we can handle it.

You don't cure AFib. You MANAGE it.

I've mentioned that we have the option of taking a pill to prevent the strokes related to AFib (there is that word *prevent* again). The question then is, how do I know if I am having AFib? Didn't I say that 90% of AFib is asymptomatic? (Why, yes. I did say that.)

Symptoms may not predict risk, but they are a great reason to begin monitoring to see if you are having any AFib. It matters. Remember, as little as five minutes of AFib, even without symptoms, will begin to increase your risk of having a stroke.

So, what are the symptoms of AFib? The most common symptoms are fast and irregular heartbeat. You may feel your heart racing for no reason. You may feel it pounding or skipping. You may be aware of an irregularity. You may simply be aware of your heart beating when you normally aren't aware of your heartbeat.

Just as commonly, AFib produces the universal heart symptoms. When you are in AFib, your heart is less efficient. Your heart is your body's pump, and when the pump is less efficient, your circulation is less efficient. Anything and everything that is waiting for blood may not work as well as it should. Thus, the universal symptoms of heart trouble relate to poor circulation.

The universal heart symptoms:
- Fatigue

- Weakness

- Tiredness

- Dizziness

- Inability to exercise or a decrease in exercise tolerance

- Breathlessness

- Lightheadedness/feeling faint

- Chest discomfort/pressure, especially with activity

- Nausea/abdominal discomfort

As you can see, these symptoms are quite non-specific. When the body is unhappy, how we feel is highly generalized. This is why measurable information, not symptoms, is so important in understanding your health and your risks.

There are many symptoms associated with AFib. When you want to know if you are having AFib, you must monitor for it.

Once you realize that you are at risk for AFib, you have to confirm it. You do that with an electro-cardiogram (ECG). When an ECG is performed, the technician will place about 10 stickers on your chest, arms, and maybe legs, and connect a bunch of wires, and then a machine will spit out a piece of graph paper with your ECG readout on it.

The diagnosis of AFib has nothing whatsoever to do with your symptoms. It is a diagnosis made by your ECG.

But remember: you can go back and forth between a normal rhythm and AFib. You can be in AFib one minute and in a normal rhythm the next. It is also possible for your heart to be irregular without it being in AFib. So, you will likely need some form of cardiac monitor that records your ECG over time to know for sure whether or not you are having AFib.

There are a variety of cardiac monitors available. The most common one is called a Holter monitor, and you wear it for a day or two while it continuously records your ECG. This is a quick, easy way to get a look at your heart's rhythm over a short period of time. A wide variety of monitors are now available to record your heart's rhythm for even longer periods of time.

One monitor in particular is worth mentioning. Medicare now covers something called an implantable cardiac monitor, designed specifically to look for AFib. This is a little microchip about the size of a paper clip that is injected under the skin (after a little numbing medicine, of course). The newest models can link to your cell phone and promptly alert your doctor if you are having AFib. The batteries last for several years.

If you want to know if you are having AFib, you have to monitor for it. There are many devices available to monitor for AFib. Work with your doctor to pick the best monitor for you.

OLD SCHOOL: We found out whether or not someone was having AFib by monitoring them for a day or two, or keeping them under observation in the hospital for a brief stay. If their AFib was not severe enough to find immediately, it was not a problem.

NEW SCHOOL: AFib can be highly intermittent and may only happen occasionally. Even brief episodes of AFib may give you a stroke, even if you don't feel it. If you want to be sure about whether you are having AFib, you have to record your heart rhythm over longer periods of time, even for years.

Good news: strokes don't happen the moment you have AFib. They typically occur weeks later. We know this from our experience with people who have had long-term monitors. This is how we found out that as little as five minutes of AFib will increase your stroke risk, but we also found that the strokes are often delayed. This makes a lot of sense. When you are in AFib, blood does not move out of the atrium smoothly. The blood pools and will start to clot. It can take some time for a clot to grow large enough to break free. When a clot breaks out of the heart, it will land in the head. That's a stroke.

The body does naturally try to reabsorb the clot. The great news is that if we discourage clots from growing, or from forming in the first place, then we win.

Strokes don't happen the minute you have AFib. This gives us the opportunity to prevent strokes if you have AFib.

Remember, you don't cure AFib. You manage it. When you have AFib, you must ask three basic questions to manage it:

1. What is the health of my heart?

2. How am I preventing strokes?

3. How do I feel?

The first question we will spend more time on later. Suffice it to say that an unhealthy heart is more likely to have AFib, and if not managed well, AFib can make a heart unhealthy.

The third question has an enormous variety of answers. This is where so much confusion comes from. Most people do not feel their AFib at all, but some people are completely incapacitated by it. There is a lot of individualization that goes along with reducing symptoms. Many of the available treatments are all about symptoms.

Many treatments for AFib will reduce symptoms or make the heart healthier, but NOT eliminate the risk for strokes.
You must always ask the second question.

When you have any AFib at all, you must ask, what am I doing to prevent strokes?
Strokes do not prevent themselves.

Procedures like cardioversions (shocking the heart to restore a regular rhythm), ablations (burning or freezing the inside of the heart to reduce the likelihood of having AFib), and pacemaker insertion can make your heart healthier. They usually improve your symptoms. They do not cure AFib. We have tried for years to cure AFib, but we have painfully learned that we can never completely guarantee that we have succeeded, and people still have strokes. Procedures may reduce the risk, but not completely eliminate it.

Even if you eliminate 99% of your AFib, you still have some AFib.

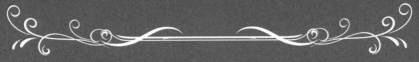

A PARABLE OF
MODERN CARDIOLOGY:

In the 1980s, we learned that a heart attack was caused by a blockage in the artery of a heart. It became quite evident that a clear artery works better than one that is blocked or partially blocked. In the 1990s and 2000s, we developed marvelous techniques to open arteries: angioplasty and stenting. We assumed that since an open artery is better than a partially blocked artery, stenting everything open must be a good idea.

Well, we were not entirely right.

Opening a blocked artery with a stent is essential in some people, but not everyone. In many people, it may be almost irrelevant. For many people, medications without a stent are just as good or even better. In some people, stenting is worse.

We developed a great new technology in stenting, but we did not yet know just how to use it. The well-meaning rush to improve blood flow did not actually cure the disease. A stent may help, but there is still a lifetime of management.

And so it is now. We are faced with a similar paradigm with procedures to cure AFib.

It is true that a heart that does not have AFib will do better than a heart that does have AFib. If you do not have AFib, you are less likely to have a stroke and less likely to have heart failure.

That does not mean that if we do a procedure to cure AFib, everything is guaranteed to be better in everyone. Just like stenting did not cure the problem of plaque buildup, a procedure to decrease the likelihood of symptomatic AFib does not necessarily make a heart healthier, decrease the risk of stroke, or decrease the chance of developing heart failure.

To be clear, ablation, especially if done at a high-quality center, is a very important tool in the management of AFib. It can be very helpful in preventing a heart from weakening in some people, and it can reduce symptoms, but not in everyone. Like stenting 20 years ago, we should not rush onto the bandwagon of a new procedure hoping for a cure, but instead we should be thoughtful about what we do, and why we are doing it.

Now, before I get pummeled by my colleagues who, like me, do these procedures, I will point out that sometimes we are successful in eliminating AFib. But, before I relax about stroke prevention, I must have some way of being sure that the AFib is truly gone. That usually requires some form of long-term monitor (like the implanted cardiac monitor, or a pacemaker).

Whatever procedures you have or don't have, you must keep asking: What am I doing to prevent strokes?

The best answer may be to do nothing, but remember: Choosing to do nothing is still a choice.

Your options for preventing a stroke when you have AFib:

1. Do nothing.

2. Implant a "closure device" that leaves a plug inside your heart to try to prevent clots from forming. (No really, we do this!)

3. Take an aspirin. (See option 1 above.)

4. Take rat poison. (Really, this is done an awful lot, and it's usually a bad idea.)

5. Take a modern stroke prevention medication.

Believe it or not, each of the preceding choices makes sense in the right situation, but the vast majority of people with AFib would be best served with a modern stroke prevention medication.

You and your doctor must choose what you are going to do to prevent strokes related to your AFib. In order to make a good choice, you need to know your personal risk of a stroke. Doing nothing is the default choice. What is the risk of that?

The risk of a stroke is not the same for everyone, but the following risks have been pretty well identified in those who have AFib:

- Age (over 65, and worse if you are over 75)

- High blood pressure

- Being a woman (woman clot better than men do!)

- A damaged heart or a history of heart failure

- Atherosclerotic disease (like a prior heart attack, or plaque in arteries)

- A prior stroke

- Diabetes

There are formulas to help add up the cumulative risk, but unless you have absolutely none of these (that is, you are a perfectly healthy young person), you have a non-trivial risk of having a stroke. With only one of the preceding risks (and you probably have more than one of them if you have AFib), then you have a 2%–5% annual risk of a stroke. If you have five or six of these risks, your risk can be 10%–15% annually.

If you choose to do nothing to prevent strokes from AFib, make sure you know what risk you are choosing to take.

I did mention that there are some invasive or even surgical procedures designed to prevent clots from forming in the heart, but these procedures are complicated, only done at experienced centers, and they are never our first choice.

Basically, in order to prevent a stroke from AFib, you simply must prevent clots from forming. We have painfully learned that we are never as perfect as we would like to think when it comes to eliminating AFib itself, so in order to prevent the stroke, you must prevent the clot.

Trying to eliminate AFib has never been enough to ensure that the risk of a stroke is gone. To prevent strokes, you must prevent clots from forming.

There is no food to eat, exercise to do, or mantra to recite that has been shown to lower the risk of stroke from AFib. There are, however, several modern medications—truly revolutionary—that are simply outstanding at preventing strokes related to AFib. They are known as direct oral anticoagulants, or DOACs. (They used to be called novel oral anticoagulants, or NOACs, but as they have been around for such a long time, the term *novel* now seems inappropriate.)

The stroke that comes from AFib is due to a clot. To prevent the stroke, you must prevent the clot. To do that, you must take a pill. Yes, we commonly call these pills "blood thinners," but I don't like that term for many reasons. First, they do nothing to change how blood flows (the physics major in me balks at the term *thinness*.) Next, the old, awful medications used to prevent blood clotting were branded as "blood thinners" so that people would take them and not question the fact that the medication was invented to kill rats. The main medicine, warfarin, was (and is) very, very hard to take safely, and it gave the term *blood thinner* a bad name. Third, there are a lot of different medications that can prevent clotting in a lot of different circumstances. They are not interchangeable.

I would rather call these medications "stroke prevention medications." Currently, there are four such medications available in the US. The most common two are Xarelto and Eliquis. One is highly effective with once-daily dosing, the other you must take twice a day. You pick.

If you have AFib, you should be on a stroke prevention medication like Xarelto or Eliquis, or have a good reason why you are not.

Yes, there are plenty of valid reasons to not take a stroke prevention medication, but make sure you have talked that through with your doctor. Not taking a stroke prevention medication is kind of like driving without a seatbelt. Yes, we all used to do it all of the time, but that doesn't make it a good idea.

Is it really that simple? I have AFib, so I take a pill to prevent strokes? Well, yes. It can be that simple. There's a pill. Take it.

OK, there must be a catch. We need to prevent clots. And the better we are at preventing clots, the more easily we can bleed.

Here's the good news: The risk of stroke without prevention is very high. The risk of significant bleeding is very low. How low? If you have AFib, you may have a 1 in 10 chance of stroke. If you take a pill to prevent that stroke, you won't have a stroke, but you'll have a 1 in 10,000 chance of a deadly bleed. You'll also have about a 2% chance of nuisance bleeding (like nosebleeds and hemorrhoids).

Human beings are hardwired to be afraid of bleeding. (Think back 100,000 years. Bleeding is bad!) But you get to decide what risks you want to take. Do you risk a lifetime of disability and brain damage, or take on a small risk of bleeding? For me, I am not overly concerned about bleeding. I have a good friend who is a gastroenterologist (a stomach specialist) who has to deal with people who have bleeding ulcers all the time. He made a very clear point when he told me, "You know, we have blood banks. We don't have brain banks." That is, what is the risk of possibly needing a transfusion versus the risk of permanent brain damage? Remember, most strokes don't kill you. They just leave you disabled.

Like I said: If it were me (or my family), I kind of like my brain. I am going to take the pill to prevent a stroke. (No, I don't have AFib yet, but I do take an aspirin daily.)

Avoid the temptation to focus on what you do NOT want to do. Instead, focus on what you DO want to prevent: strokes.
I'll say it again: Choosing to do nothing is still a choice. If you choose that, make sure you've thought it through.

In the old days, we used to use a medication called warfarin to prevent strokes in people who had AFib. Warfarin was created in 1948 (it's a baby boomer med!) as a way to kill rats by making them bleed to death. It is an astonishing drug that would never get FDA approval today because we never know how it will affect you. No one ever knows the dose they will need. It is not what we would call a direct anticoagulant. It works indirectly by altering the metabolism of things we eat that may or may not influence how well our liver works, blah blah blah...

It is an awful drug.

How awful? In our best research trials, with weekly blood tests, we can only get the drug in an effective range about half of the time. The rest of the time we are either underdosing, which leaves people unprotected from strokes, or we are overdosing, making people bleed. Half the time we are off, even when we try hard. And people bleed. And they stroke.

Yet, despite all of that, taking warfarin is still a whole lot better than doing nothing. Don't underestimate how bad it is to have a stroke.

If you have a mechanical heart valve replacement, we still use warfarin, but that's about the only case in which it is used. If your doctor recommends it, ask for him or her to consider learning about drugs that were developed in this century.

OLD SCHOOL: Anticoagulation is hard. All we had was warfarin (trade name Coumadin), which was first developed in 1948 to kill rats. It works by changing the metabolism of what we eat, so different foods are always changing things. It means you have to get constant blood tests for the rest of your life. Half the time we either prescribed too much or too little of it. Your dose could randomly change. If you were bleeding, we had to try to reverse the effect of the medication with a different medication that would take more than a day to make a difference. It took some convincing that taking warfarin was worth it.

NEW SCHOOL: Stroke prevention with a 21st-century medication is easy. It works directly on the blood, so the dosing is well known. No blood tests are needed. It reliably works. You can eat anything you want. You bleed a lot less. If you have to, you can turn off the blood thinning effect promptly. Why exactly would you not protect yourself from a stroke if you have AFib?

The AFib summary:

- AFib is common and it is largely due to age.

- If you want to know if you have AFib, you must use some form of cardiac monitor.

- Your symptoms have no correlation to your risk of a stroke.

- If you do nothing, your stroke risk is high.

- If you have AFib, you can take a pill to prevent strokes.

There are no absolutes. Nothing is perfect. Everyone is unique. As I said in the beginning, the first step in preventing strokes is to have a relationship with a good doctor to help you navigate these things and help you make the choices that make the most sense for you.

NOTES:

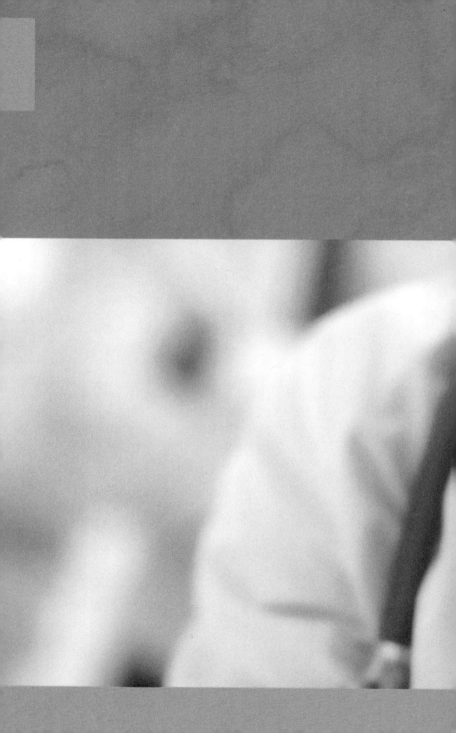

CHAPTER 5

HEALTHY BRAIN? HEALTHY HEART.

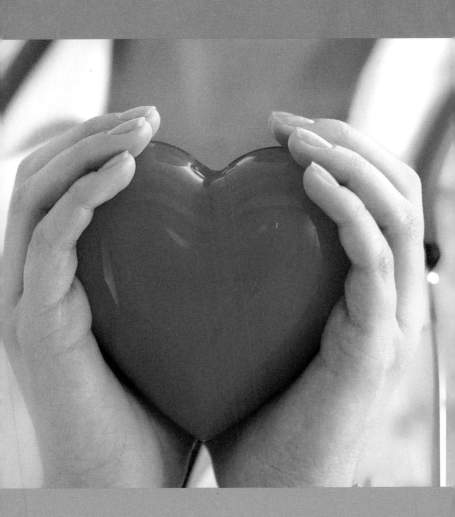

I used to drive a '69 VW Beetle. It eventually stopped running right. I took it to the mechanic. "What's wrong with it?" I asked. "It's got engine trouble," he said. No, really?

My mechanic telling me that my car had engine trouble was about as useful as a doctor telling you that you have "heart failure." If your heart is not running as well as your body needs it to, then your heart is failing you. That may be the most important thing you are ever told, and the most useless. If your heart isn't working right, it definitely matters *why*.

If your heart isn't working as efficiently as it should, then blood doesn't flow as well as your body wants it to. More importantly, blood doesn't flow to your brain as well as your brain needs it to.

As we said earlier, a stroke is a cerebrovascular accident. That is, brain damage from not getting blood to the brain. Even worse, vascular dementia is what happens to the brain when it chronically does not get adequate blood flow.

Vascular dementia is the chronic brain damage that results from inadequate or interrupted blood flow to the brain.
The brain does not suck blood up from the body. The heart pumps it there. If you want to

get adequate blood flow to the brain, you have to keep the heart working well.

Healthy brains require healthy hearts. You must maintain good blood flow to the brain. We need to keep our pumps working. Fortunately, there are only so many ways that a heart can be damaged or become inefficient. We know who the usual suspects are, and we know how to round them up. Most of these things, in fact, are entirely predictable.

There is (almost) no such thing as heart disease. It is just natural aging. Don't get me wrong. Mother Nature always wins, but when it comes to the heart, aging is largely predictable, measurable, and manageable.

Hearts naturally become less efficient over time, even if you don't have overt heart disease. If your body or brain needs more blood than your heart is giving it, then you have inefficient circulation. This doesn't mean you have had a heart attack. It doesn't mean you have heart damage. It doesn't have to mean you have heart failure.

OLD SCHOOL: Heart failure means you are swollen and breathless with a weak heart, and you need to see a cardiologist who will give you pills to breathe better. Dementia means that your brain doesn't work. You should see a neurologist, who can tell you what to expect.

NEW SCHOOL: The heart works to support the brain. When the heart is not working well, blood flow suffers, and the brain will eventually suffer, leading to strokes, brain damage, and dementia. To protect the brain, you have to understand the health of your heart and your circulation, and do everything you can to keep blood flowing to your brain.

Your brain depends upon your heart's efficiency.

To understand the health and efficiency of your heart, it is helpful to think about the most common factors related to aging that affect the heart and lead to heart disease. Everyone has at least three things that will affect the heart over time:

1. **BLOCKED ARTERIES** (atherosclerosis, heart attacks, coronary artery disease)
2. **HIGH BLOOD PRESSURE** (hypertension)

3. **HEART RATE AND RHYTHM** (slow heart rate, also called bradycardia and AFib)

Recall from our chapter on aging that everyone gets atherosclerosis with age. Everyone can have hypertension with age. Everyone can have a slower and irregular heartbeat with age. (Heart valves can also be a problem, but this is a more variable, individual issue that you'll need to talk to your cardiologist about.) Understanding the processes of aging gives us the opportunity to stay healthy. Not only can we prevent strokes, we can manage our aging and largely prevent heart failure as well. Preventing heart failure is very good for the brain (and the heart!).

So, to keep a heart and brain healthy, it is useful to think of the aging-related factors that will affect you.

 Blocked Arteries

The coronary arteries are the arteries that feed the heart. The heart pumps blood to every part of the body, including itself. The coronary arteries sit on top of the heart like a crown (that's how they get their name, like "coronation"— get it?). We already mentioned that 100,000 heartbeats a day cause a lot of wear and tear on arteries. Age leads to chronic vascular inflammation, which leads to plaque growth.

The coronary arteries that feed the heart are actually pretty small—barely more than ¼ inch (3–4 mm) across. It does not take all that much plaque to begin blocking an artery. When a coronary artery is blocked, the heart muscle downstream waiting for blood starts to die. When it happens suddenly, we call it a heart attack.

You do not have to have a heart attack to damage the heart this way. If your arteries are chronically blocked, or partially blocked, you can slowly starve your heart muscle and damage it. The net result is a weak heart muscle.

This is what most people think of as heart disease—blocked arteries and damaged heart muscle. If enough muscle is damaged, the heart becomes weak. A weak heart cannot pump blood to the brain well.

Blocked coronary arteries are the traditional cause of a weak heart and heart failure. You can have a weak heart without dramatic symptoms (see the universal heart symptoms in the preceding chapter). You can have partially blocked arteries with no symptoms at all.

If you don't want a weak heart from blocked coronary arteries, then don't get coronary artery disease. That means don't let plaque build up. The same steps that prevent plaque in the carotid arteries prevent plaque everywhere. Take a statin. Take something to prevent clots. Funny, preventing heart attacks is simple compared to preventing strokes.

② *High Blood Pressure*

Age stiffens arteries. Arteries are the pipes that carry blood. Stiffer pipes mean higher blood pressure. Higher blood pressure means more cardiac work. More cardiac work means the heart muscle will become thicker and stiffer. A thick, stiff heart can be very inefficient.

Before blood is pumped out of the heart and into the body, the heart has to fill with blood. The heart must relax in order to fill with blood. But high blood pressure and age makes a heart stiff, which means it has trouble relaxing to fill. If the heart doesn't fill with blood, there's no blood to pump out, no matter how strong the heart is.

The issue is blood *flow*. We need blood to flow to carry oxygen to the brain. A stiff heart has trouble generating good blood flow.

You see, blood pressure is a number, not a disease. The issue is the health of our heart and our arteries.

Blood flow matters more than blood pressure. The challenge, of course, is that we measure blood pressure. We can't easily measure blood flow. But our blood pressure represents how hard it is to maintain blood flow, how stiff our arteries are, and how much work our heart is doing. If we chronically overwork our heart, we will have heart failure from a stiff heart due to blood pressure.

High blood pressure will lead to a stiff heart and heart failure, even though the heart may be strong.
So, if you don't want to have heart failure from high blood pressure, be aggressive in preventing the aging of your arteries (exercise, don't smoke, reduce salt) and talk with your doctor about medication to control blood pressure and maintain vascular health.

(3) Heart Rate and Rhythm

It is pretty well known that we don't want to get plaque in our arteries because it can damage our heart, and we don't want to have untreated high blood pressure because that can damage the heart. What is less well known is that we don't want our heart to beat too fast, too slow, or too irregular as that can create problems for our heart as well.

Heart *rate* is also called "pulse." It is the number of times per minute that our heart beats. A typical, average heart rate is 60–80 beats per minute (bpm). Heart rate and blood pressure are not the same thing. For the most part, they are independent.

Heart *rhythm* is the pattern in which the heart beats. A normal rhythm is called a sinus rhythm. An abnormal rhythm is called an arrhythmia. The most common abnormal rhythm is AFib. AFib can be fast (have a high rate) or be slow (have a low rate). The pattern of AFib is always irregular regardless of the rate.

Recall: AFib is very common if we live long enough. When most people first have AFib, the heart tends to race. That is, the heart rate is high, and the heart beats really fast. If a heart beats fast continuously for weeks or months, it will weaken and dilate or stretch out and enlarge. That will give you heart failure and poor blood flow.

A continuously fast heart rate can cause a heart to weaken and dilate. This can happen with AFib.

Less commonly, the irregularity alone will weaken the heart, even if it is not beating too fast. These are the folks who may benefit from aggressively preventing AFib. Irregularity always makes blood flow less efficiently, even if the heart is not weak.

Fast heart rates are a problem. Irregular heart rhythms are a problem. But what may be the most common problem is a slow heart rate. How much blood we circulate is known as our *cardiac output*. Cardiac output is simply how much blood our heart pumps with each heartbeat times how many heartbeats we have: Cardiac output = (volume of a heartbeat) × (heart rate).

Our blood flow depends heavily (but not exclusively) on our heart rate.
When we are young, our heart rate may reflect fitness. All my athletic friends, especially the runners, are fond of bragging about how slow their heart rate is. The bicyclists are even worse (because they both brag and wear spandex).

When we are fit, our body, especially our muscles, are very efficient and do not need much blood flow. Since they do not need much blood flow, the heart does not have to circulate much, especially when we are resting. Thus, young athletes can have very slow heart rates.

Good for them.

When they get older, the heart rate naturally slows down *just because they are older*, not because they got more fit.

When we are young, the heart rate can be slow because we are athletic. When we are older, the heart rate is slow because we are older, not because we are athletic.

Athletes with slow hearts often have a lot of trouble when they are over 65 because their hearts are too slow for what their bodies need. First, think of that formula: Cardiac output = (volume of a heart beat) × (heart rate). If the rate goes down, the volume has to go up to maintain a steady blood flow. If the volume goes up too much, the heart will stretch, and that leads to heart failure.

A slow heart can lead to heart failure.
Even simpler than that, if your heart is too slow, you are simply not circulating as much blood. This is a very important point that is often overlooked. A slow heart rate means less blood is flowing. That means the brain gets less blood. Over time, the brain slowly suffers. This is one of the key drivers of senility, or vascular dementia.

A heart rate that is too slow can be a cause of vascular dementia.
The major trouble with this is that the changes can happen very gradually. No one notices until you realize that your spouse is just not the same person they used to be. It can take years.

OLD SCHOOL: A slow heart rate is a good sign of fitness and health. Unless someone has fainted, you never need to worry about a slow heart rate.

NEW SCHOOL: Aging alone will slow a heart. Blood flow depends upon our heart beating, and if it beats too slowly, the heart and brain will suffer. A slow heart from age alone can lead to heart failure, brain damage, and dementia. A slow heart in a young person may be desirable, but in an older person, it will eventually be a problem.

We did mention that a slow heart rate also encourages AFib. AFib creates another issue. When you have AFib (and currently 6 million Americans are in AFib all of the time), it is important to control the heart rate. If the heart rate is too fast, the heart can weaken. So, we use all sorts of medications to slow down the AFib.

The problem is that AFib is irregularly irregular. The vast majority of the time we may have a perfectly reasonable heart rate, but on occasion, the heart skips beats and *pauses*. During a pause, the heart is not beating at all. We all have the occasional skipped beats, or pauses. The pause is usually less than two seconds long, and we rarely notice it. In AFib, many people experience longer pauses that happen more frequently. If you have a three- to four-second pause without a heartbeat, you might faint (without warning). What's more, that's three to four seconds without good blood flow to your brain. You can only do that so much before your brain suffers.

The heart can pause, and not beat, especially when we are in AFib.
This can happen even if we have a normal or fast tempo most of the time. You might be surprised at how often your heart is not beating. It's not a good thing, and you often won't feel it.

If you have too slow a heart rate, or too many pauses without a heartbeat, you will damage your brain from lack of blood flow.
For better or worse, the brain damage is usually subtle at first. True brain damage takes a lot of time. This does give us plenty of time to recognize the issue and prevent problems.
There is no pill for a slow heart rate. There is no diet or exercise that will restore the tempo of your heart when it is too slow. You can, however, get a pacemaker when you need one.

The problems from a slow heart can be prevented with a pacemaker.
Nowadays, pacemakers are easy. It is a quick outpatient procedure that involves little more

than some local numbing medicine and a few stitches. Yes, I implant pacemakers, so I am biased. I know how easy it is to get one, and I know how much better people can feel when they have one. I know that it is easier to get a pacemaker than a root canal, and it's covered by insurance. As a matter of fact, all of my 100-year-old patients, except one, have a pacemaker. I have a lot of 100-year-old patients. My oldest patient is still sharp as a tack at 106, and as I said before, she still complains that no one will dance with her.

We all want to keep a healthy brain. To keep a healthy brain, we must keep a healthy heart. To keep a healthy heart, we must avoid or prevent heart damage. We must not let plaque build up in our coronary arteries, which will starve the heart of blood and damage it. We must not allow our arteries to get so stiff that our blood pressure rises and overworks our hearts so that it no longer pumps blood well.

We have to remember that age changes things. Our bodies work differently at 70 than they did at 17. We need to keep blood flowing to our brains. We need to have a strong heartbeat, and we need to have enough of them.

In the final chapters we will talk about how our doctors can help us, and how we can help ourselves.

NOTES:

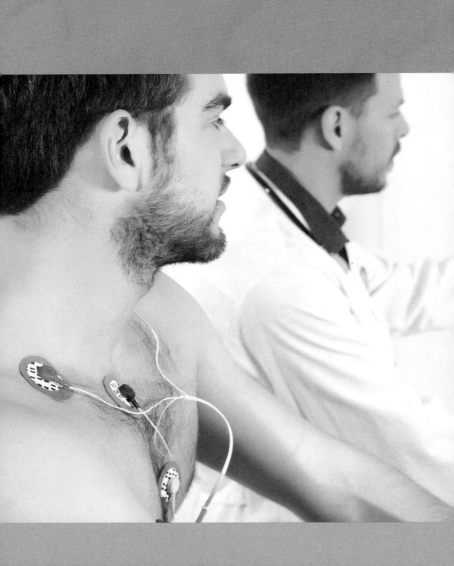

CHAPTER 6

TRUST, BUT VERIFY

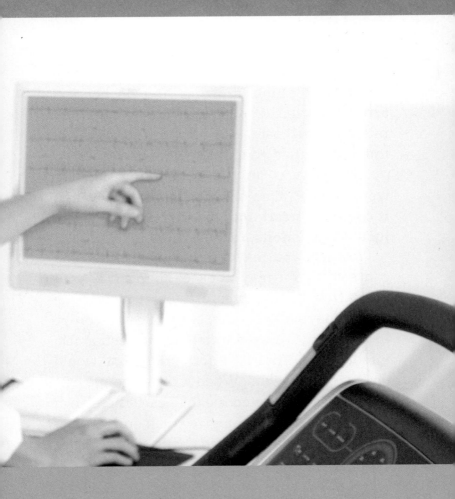

I was in college in the 1980s when Ronald Reagan was president. I can't say I remember everything that happened in college, but I do remember my favorite Reagan quote: "Trust, but verify."

Granted, he was talking about Soviets, but it is wisdom that applies very well to understanding our own health. We need to verify that we are as healthy as we think we are.

Heart and vascular disease is a silent killer, but it is not invisible. We can see it.
Remember, symptoms do not predict risk. You do not feel plaque growing. You do not feel arteries stiffen. You do not feel irregular or missed heartbeats. Not at first, anyway. Not until you've had your stroke or heart attack.

When I was an intern at Johns Hopkins, we had rules. One of those rules was: **When it comes to heart and vascular disease, don't just ask questions, take pictures.**

You see, you may not feel plaque, but you can see it. You may not feel changes to your heart from higher pressure, but you can see it. You may not feel AFib, but you can record it. In the Navy, we used to talk about "actionable intelligence." That is, information that would change what we did. When it comes to preventing strokes and protecting the heart, there are a few basic tests that can give you a great deal of actionable intelligence and change what we do.

TALES
· FROM THE ·
OLD DAYS

When I was an intern at The Johns Hopkins Hospital, I used to drive my chief resident nuts. (Sorry about that, Billy!) At Hopkins, there was a general philosophy that we did not want to leave any question unanswered. We did not like to have any diagnostic uncertainty if there was a test that could be done.

The problem is that not all diagnostic tests are benign, let alone useful. I used to challenge my chief with the notion that I would not place a patient at risk with an invasive test if the outcome did not change management. In other words, I would only perform a test if the results of those tests would meaningfully change how we treated someone.

Today, there are so many tests available for so many conditions. Before we agree to a test, we should know, what are we going to do with the results? If the test results don't change anything, then why do it?

Additionally, if there are treatment options available (like taking a pill to prevent a stroke if you have AFib), and when there is diagnostic uncertainty, then you really need to ask what tests are available to you to best guide your therapy.

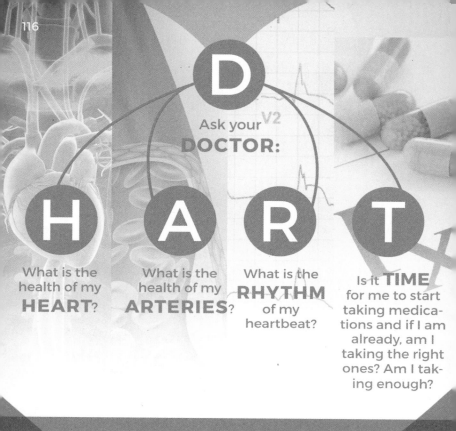

D

Ask your V2
DOCTOR:

H What is the health of my **HEART**?

A What is the health of my **ARTERIES**?

R What is the **RHYTHM** of my heartbeat?

T Is it **TIME** for me to start taking medications and if I am already, am I taking the right ones? Am I taking enough?

The first challenge is finding a doctor to work with. I'll leave that to you. The next challenge is learning to work with your doctor. For better or worse, doctors in the past were often taught to respond to symptoms, whereas younger doctors are taught how to click on their computers to fill out the electronic medical record (EMR).

What you need to do is help your doctor answer those questions we outlined in the very beginning in the Foxhall Formula, or D-HART strategy.

If you want to know how healthy something is, look at it.

Since so many doctors and so many EMR systems are driven by symptoms, before you go to your doctor, take some time to think to yourself about how you feel.

- Can you run uphill really fast, forever, without becoming breathless?

- Have you ever felt, or been worried, that your heartbeat may have been irregular?

- Have you ever been lightheaded or felt faint?

If you answered "no" to all of these questions, then you are, in fact, Superman or Wonder Woman. The rest of us mortals have limits. Even Olympic athletes and Navy Seals eventually reach a limit. Presumably, you can get breathless and you have wondered about an irregular heartbeat, and you may have felt faint. So, congratulations, you have the common symptoms shortness of breath, palpitations, and syncope.

Symptoms do not predict risk, but they do validate an evaluation of your heart and vascular health.

If you go to a doctor who practices preventive cardiology and say, "I want to know my heart's health and stroke risk," they can embark on a

TRUST, BUT VERIFY

systematic evaluation for you. You don't need a reason to want to prevent strokes.

More commonly, a primary care provider, who has been allotted no more than six minutes to see you and fill out your EMR, will need a reason for you to get an evaluation. Fine. Tell them that you get short of breath when you run hard, and you want to know that it's safe to exercise, so you want to have an evaluation.

OLD SCHOOL: In truly ancient times, doctors were free to order whatever diagnostic tests they thought were in the best interest of their patient.

NEW SCHOOL: Many health care providers operate under protocols dictated by the mandatory reporting requirements of the EMRs. Fortunately, current Medicare policies are quite thorough in covering medical testing, but your provider may be required to link a specific diagnosis to a test. In the absence of well-defined diagnoses, symptoms, such as breathlessness, chest discomfort, palpitations, dizziness, or syncope, will appropriately drive medical testing. Feel free to tell your clinic, medical home, or primary care provider what symptoms you have.

Anyone can examine you, check your blood pressure, get an ECG, and order basic lab work (blood tests). If any of those things are less than absolutely perfect, then that is also a reason to go forward with a closer look at your heart, circulation, and risk for stroke.

Remember, strokes come from problems with circulation, not problems with the brain, so you will want some pictures of your heart and circulation.

A brain scan will only tell you if your brain has already been damaged. It does not tell you about future risks or how to prevent future strokes.

The first thing to know is the health of your heart. That can be verified with an ultrasound of your heart (an echocardiogram, or echo). The echo will tell you if you have heart damage already. It will tell you if your heart is weak or dilated. It will tell you if you have overworked your heart. It will tell you if your blood pressure control has been adequate. It will tell you if your heart is stiff and inefficient. It will tell you if your atrium has been stretched out already and if you are at high risk for AFib.

My goodness. An echo tells you an awful lot. When I meet a new patient, I will look at their echo before I even say hello. It saves a lot of time if I know the health of their heart first.

It is important that you and your doctor know what the echo is telling you. Ask questions like, how strong is my heart? Has my heart been damaged? Has my blood pressure been adequately controlled? Am I at risk of getting AFib?

An echo, or ultrasound of the heart, is an important, easy way to know about the health of your heart and your stroke risk.

Of course, looking good when you are sitting still is one thing. You want to know how you look when you are up and moving—when you are under stress. There are a lot of ways you can test the heart. There are a lot of different types of stress tests. But, if you want to know how well your circulation is working, the best way to do that is to watch you work.

We call the test a stress echocardiogram. Yes, it is a type of stress test, but I prefer to think of it as a functional assessment. How is your function? How do your heart and circulation respond to activity, exercise, work, or stress? What does your heart rate do? What does your blood pressure do? How is your oxygen level? Do you have AFib when you exercise? Are you likely to have a heart attack? How is the function of your coronary arteries?

If you can walk, you can walk in front of your doctor on a treadmill. It is generally better for your doctor to watch you walk (rather than an anonymous technician). That way, your doctor sees what happens to you. There is no "passing" or "failing" a stress test. Everybody reaches a limit. No one beats the machine. It can always go faster. Your doctor, if they are watching, can tell you what it is that makes you reach your limit.

There are a lot of different heart tests. They all look for different things in different ways. They all have uses at different times. Ultimately, how your heart WORKS FOR YOU is the most important thing. All you need to do in order to know is to look.

A simple, reliable way to know exactly how your heart works is to have your doctor watch you exercise. This can easily be done with a stress echocardiogram.

Again, all you have to do is walk. I have 90-year-olds who get up and walk on a treadmill for me. Some of them go faster than people a third their age. It's amazing how much you can find out about your heart and circulation if you look.

A quick story to illustrate: A woman asked me to see her 70-year-old husband because he felt that he got short of breath when walking.

He had a great team of cardiologists at a wonderful academic medical center. He had a pacemaker. The pacemaker specialist checked his pacemaker and assured him that it was working normally. He had an echo, and the head of the echo lab assured him that his echo was normal. He had two different tests to image his coronary arteries and test their blood flow. Those two doctors also reported normal results. The conclusion: your heart is not the cause of your breathlessness. Have a nice day.

His wife, naturally tired of hearing him complain about being out of breath all of the time, brought him to me. I asked him simply, "You say you get out of breath when you are walking. Did anyone watch you walk?"

Well, of course not.

So we put him on a treadmill (which most cardiologists are told is meaningless in patients with pacemakers). You see, you can program a pacemaker to speed up when you walk. When we are walking, we are supposed to have a faster heart rate. (How else do we increase blood flow?) How do you know if you have programmed the pacemaker well enough? Well, you can TRUST that the programming is right, or you can VERIFY it.

Sure enough, his heart beat 60 times a minute when he was sitting still. It beat 60 times a minute when he started walking. It beat 60 times a minute no matter how fast the treadmill was going. And he was short of breath. You try running with a heart rate of 60. We reprogrammed his pacemaker while he was on the treadmill so that the pacemaker would better recognize when he was exercising. The pacemaker then increased his heart rate. His cardiac output increased, and his breathlessness was gone. Amazing. (Having dropped out of graduate school for astrophysics, I can assure you, this is not rocket science. It's just attention to detail.)

Trust, but verify. If you want to know your heart's function, test it.

Remember, we need our hearts to work well if we want to protect the brain. So the next thing to ask is, how regular is my heartbeat? We keep harping on the point that irregular heartbeats matter. AFib is common. AFib is usually asymptomatic or minimally symptomatic at first. So, you need to verify whether you are having AFib or not. To do that, you need to do some form of monitoring of your heart's rhythm.

Tell your doctor that you have felt an irregular heartbeat, or whatever it is you have felt. Maybe you felt your heart skip. Maybe you felt it race. Maybe you felt it pound. Maybe you felt intermittent pressure or intermittent breathlessness. Maybe you felt a flutter. Different people perceive their heartbeats in different ways. The symptoms may be trivial or alarming, but either way, it's not the symptoms that count. It's the rhythm and rate of your heart that counts. The symptoms will just help you work with your doctor to figure out the best way to study your heart.

There are a lot of different ways to monitor your heart to look for irregular heartbeats and AFib. Your doctor may give you the 24-hour Holter monitor. You may get a two-week or a four-week monitor. You can buy your own monitor. The new smart watches help (but they are far from perfect).

The best monitor is the implantable cardiac monitor. That's the paperclip-sized microchip your doctor can insert under your skin. Those never miss AFib, even if it's asymptomatic.

Trust, but verify. If you are at risk for AFib, or think you are having AFib, you need to monitor for it.

Work with your doctor until you are both satisfied that you know exactly how regular your heart rhythm is. Know whether or not you have AFib. Know if your heart is too slow or too fast. Know if you are having pauses. Know how often you have pauses, how long they are, and if they matter. Ask if it is time for a new medication. Ask if it is time for a pacemaker. All of these things can be known if you look for the answers. Ask your doctor to help.

And what about those arteries? That's kind of easy. If you want to know how healthy your arteries are, then look. We no longer rely just on blood tests. Hypothetically, we don't treat cholesterol anymore. Well, at least not just for the sake of the number. Our guidelines suggest that we treat risk. That is to say, when your risk for having a vascular event (a stroke or heart attack) is high enough, then you can be started on vascular protective medications (that is, statin therapy and something to prevent clots).

We have several formulas for calculating risk of heart attack and stroke. In all of the formulas (also called "risk calculators") age is one of the variables. The higher your age, the higher your risk. So, if you live long enough, according to the guidelines, everyone is supposed to take a statin eventually. Do you really have to? Or better yet, are you taking enough? Why do people with normal cholesterol still have heart attacks and strokes? How do I know if I am growing plaque? How do I know if my treatment is adequate?

If you want to know, look. The simplest way is to ask for a high-resolution ultrasound of your arteries, specifically your carotid arteries. Your carotid arteries are ideal for this. They are easy to see, and they are important, as they are often the first arteries to show any evidence of vascular aging (that is, plaque growth).

Our heart pumps blood up, straight to the brain first. The carotid arteries fork right below our skull (one branch goes to our brain, the other our scalp). This fork in the artery generates turbulent blood flow. This turbulence promotes injury and inflammation, so plaque typically grows there first.

Plaque is not something that sticks to an artery. It grows within the wall of the artery. That's why ultrasound is so good at seeing it. Ultrasound can see through the wall of the artery to see how much plaque you have growing.

A high-resolution carotid ultrasound is a great way to verify your arterial health.

Why a high-resolution scan? Well, it's not really about the ultrasound, it's about how the information is interpreted. In ancient times (like a few years ago), the only treatment we had for plaque in arteries was surgery. We would operate on a carotid artery to cut out the plaque. But this was only helpful if there was so much plaque that the artery was at least 70% blocked. Anything less than 50% blocked would never cause flow to slow down and would never be operated on. Therefore, carotid ultrasounds that showed 0–49% blockage used to be interpreted as normal.

There is a whole lot of difference between having zero plaque and having so much plaque that it blocks 49% of the artery. To this day, I see reports on carotid arteries that read, "0–49% blockage." That tells me almost nothing.

OLD SCHOOL: We used to only look at a carotid ultrasound after someone had a stroke. The idea apparently was to see why it happened so maybe we could help prevent a second stroke. In days gone by, the only intervention was a surgical one. Since no one with less than a 50% blockage needed surgery, arteries with anywhere from 0–49% blockage were called "normal."

NEW SCHOOL: We would rather prevent the first stroke, not just wait for it to happen and only prevent the second stroke. Also, there is nothing normal about an artery that has so much plaque that it is blocked 49%. In fact, several recent studies have shown a major reduction in the risk of stroke if we more thoroughly prevent clots when someone has a 50% blockage in a carotid artery, even if they are asymptomatic. In the new school, arterial disease is treated with medications, not surgery (except in extreme cases).

A quality carotid ultrasound can tell you about how much plaque you have (your plaque burden). If you have had an ultrasound in the past, you can compare it to see if your plaque burden has increased. This is enormously helpful.

You can compare your carotid artery ultrasound to previous studies to see if you have an increase in plaque in your arteries.

If you have an increase in plaque, then you have an opportunity to do something about it. It is natural for plaque to grow, but you can prevent that. You prevent plaque growth to prevent strokes.

What can be done? If your cholesterol is too high, work on it. If your diabetes is not well controlled, work on it. If you smoke, stop. If you're not taking any meds, you need to start! If you are on meds, you need to do more or something different. This is where you can gain a lot by working with your doctor.

If you have an increase in plaque, there are many things you can do to prevent further plaque growth.

Statin medications prevent most plaque growth in most people. But there are some people (not many, really) who cannot tolerate them. There are some new medications that work to prevent plaque growth as well. Remember, the goal is to not have a stroke. The goal is not to have nice cholesterol numbers. You prevent strokes by preventing plaque growth. You aren't going to know if you are preventing plaque growth unless you look. Fortunately, it's easy to look.

OLD SCHOOL: We treated cholesterol. We measured blood tests, and declared success when the numbers were good.

NEW SCHOOL: We set our goal to be the prevention of strokes. We adjust treatment based on plaque burden, not just cholesterol. If you are growing more plaque, even if you have good cholesterol numbers, then we consider other options to improve the health of your arteries and prevent strokes.

As we said in the very beginning of this book, one of the first things that you can do to prevent strokes and dementia is to have a good relationship with a doctor. That doctor, possibly with the help of a cardiologist, can work with you to understand your heart and vascular health. Aging of your heart and circulation is going to happen, but the aging process is largely predictable, measurable, and manageable. The measurements are the tests that you can have done with your doctor's assistance.

In my practice, regular patients typically will have an echocardiogram and a stress echocardiogram eventually, and at some point a carotid ultrasound and some form of cardiac monitoring. When we have done this, we know just about everything we need to know about their heart and circulation.

We know if they have atherosclerotic disease and if it is adequately treated. We know what we have to do to prevent heart attacks and strokes related to plaque growth. We know if it's time for a medicine to prevent plaque growth and if we're doing a good enough job.

We know if they have hypertensive (high blood pressure–related) heart and vascular disease. We know if it is controlled well and we know how to treat it. We know how to prevent them from having heart failure and poor circulation to the brain. We know which medications are helpful, and if they are adequately dosed.

We know if their marching band has an unreliable drum major—if their natural pacemaker is too slow or unreliable (see Chapter 3). We know if they are having AFib. We know when it's time to consider procedures for AFib or if it's time for a pacemaker. We know if it's time to take a medication to prevent clots and prevent strokes.

The health of your heart and circulation is a knowable thing. But you have to ask the questions.

In short, your entire cardiovascular risk, your risk of a stroke, a heart attack, heart failure, or vascular dementia is something that can be known. These problems are preventable, and knowing your health gives you options on how to prevent them.

You aren't expected to do this alone. In fact, you really can't. Your doctor can help you—but you may have to take the initiative.

You may have to be the one who asks the questions. If nothing else, remember the Foxhall Formula, D-HART: "Doctor, how are my Heart, my Arteries, my Rhythm? Is it Time to change medications?"

Ultimately, it's your heart, your brain, your life. You ask the questions.

NOTES:

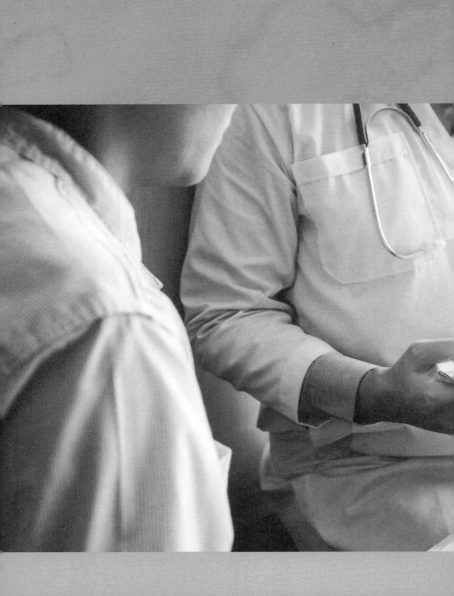

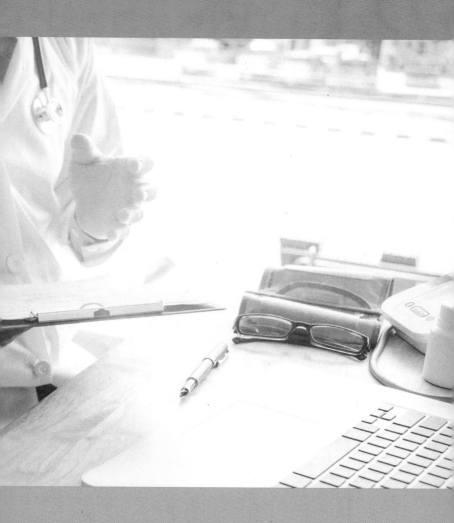

CHAPTER 7

NAVIGATING (WITH) YOUR DOCTOR

When I was a kid, my dad drove everywhere. He never asked for directions. He seemed to have a vague sense of where we were supposed to go and how to get there, and then drove in that general direction. There was no technology to guide him and few roads to choose from, and for the most part, we seemed to do OK.

I always like to look at a map first. I like to know my goal, have a plan, and understand that there is more than one way to get to where I want to be. I use technology to help guide me along the way. I have contingencies and maintain flexibility.

My kids seem to need technology just to know where they are. They think of some destination, not really knowing where it is or how to get there, and again rely on technology to give them directions each step of the way, and they are often stumped when confronted with an unexpected obstacle.

So it is with doctors.

How your doctor approaches your health is often a reflection of their generation and how they were trained. When I was in med school, 70 was considered old. Much of our technology (especially imaging) was just being developed. There were few treatment options and thus limited expectations.

Regional and institutional variations also affect how doctors are trained. Doctors tend to do things the way they were taught. How things are done in Baltimore is remarkably different than how they are done in Washington. That doesn't mean one of us is wrong.

Medicine is both an art and a science. There is no single way to practice.

Additionally, most doctors do not change their practice patterns all that much once they are more than five years out of training. That means doctors do not tend to evolve.

But medicine advances, and we are always learning more. I routinely tell my patients that I want to see them regularly. I tell them, "Come back in a year. Even if you don't change, sometimes I get smarter."

Doctors can get smarter, and they often learn when their patients inspire them.

As I said in the beginning of the book, the most important first step is to have a relationship with a physician. A primary care physician, or internist, is like the queen on a chessboard. She is the most useful piece. An internist can know anything, but they can't know everything (with the possible exception of Dr. Thomas). The best internists have a cadre of specialists within their community to help them.

What your internist has likely never been taught is this: Heart and vascular disease is a part of natural aging. You have to anticipate it, measure it, and manage it. As a patient, you can help your doctor help you. But remember, working with your doctor is like driving with someone. How you give directions changes based on whether you are driving with your parents, your spouse, or your kids. Your doctor already has a way of seeing things.

We screen for cancer. We vaccinate against infections. We prevent heart and vascular disease. That last part is the new way of looking at things.

All primary care doctors are used to screening for cancer because early detection of cancer allows for earlier treatment, more options, and better outcomes. Not everyone will get cancer, but everyone will age. Everyone will develop changes to their heart and circulation. Everyone will have a risk of stroke and heart failure. In fact, more people die of blood clots than breast cancer, and the most common cause of death for women with breast cancer is still heart disease.

And that's great.

That means many more cancer patients are dying of "old age," not their cancer. The key is, we don't want to die of old age prematurely, and we don't want strokes or dementia. So, you have to know your own heart and vascular health. You won't know until you find out.

So, who should have their heart and vascular health evaluated? Everyone.

Remember, we are not screening for heart disease. We are evaluating heart and vascular health. Everyone changes. The question is not whether you have heart disease, but how far along you are, and what you can do about it.

First question: Who should have their heart and vascular health evaluated? Answer: Everyone. Next question: When? Well, that depends on the person. The traditional approach is to identify risk factors. The major risk factors for atherosclerotic disease are family history, age, diabetes, smoking, high blood pressure, and high cholesterol.

The problem with this line of thinking is that it implies that if we eliminate the risk factors, we eliminate the disease. Remember, it's not a disease. It's a natural process. So, instead of just asking what are my risk factors, we can ask, what do my genetics tell me, and how much has my circulation aged?

Genetic testing sounds really exciting, but the genes behind vascular aging are numerous. The best, easiest genetic test is to ask, how is the health of my family?

I usually ask my patients to tell me about the health of their parents. What do you really know? "Well, dad died of old age." (Really? How old, 70?) "And mom had dementia." (She probably had AFib and multiple strokes.) "Well, they didn't take care of themselves." Fine.

Then you have a preview of what your genetics have in store for you if you don't take care of yourself.

Whatever age your parent (or sibling for that matter) showed any sign of having heart or vascular disease (that is, heart attack, heart failure, stroke, dementia, death), you need to realize that their circulation started to change 10 years before that.

That's when you need to start looking.

Think of the earliest age that a family member had evidence of heart or vascular disease. Consider studying your own heart and vascular health when you are 10 years younger than that.

You can help your doctor do this with you. Analyze your family history. Discuss with your doctor the things that will accelerate your aging (like high blood pressure, high cholesterol, and diabetes). Figure out at what age you need to verify your heart and vascular health. (Remember: Trust, but verify.)

In practice, current guidelines suggest we start thinking about heart and vascular health at age 40. By age 50, if you haven't sat down with a doctor to discuss your heart and vascular health, then you really should. And by 65 you really need to start verifying your health.

We should start to verify our heart and vascular health when we are 10 years younger than the youngest family member with heart or vascular problems, or at least by age 65.

After you've asked your doctor about the health of your heart and circulation, follow up by asking, how do we know? We all reach the point when we need to verify our heart and vascular health. There are a lot of ways to do this. This is where regional variation, available resources, and institutional expertise and experience come in. There is no single way to do this, but there are some themes.

Recall the D-HART strategy (the Foxhall Formula):

- Ask your Doctor about the health of your Heart and Arteries, your Rhythm, and whether it's Time for medication changes.

- Why? Knowing these things will let you know how you can prevent strokes and dementia (and heart failure for that matter). We want to have testing done that will lead to actionable information.

Testing is an essential part of knowing your heart and vascular health. For every test ordered, you should ask in advance, what am I going to do with this information? Will it change what I do?

NAVIGATING (WITH) YOUR DOCTOR

So, it can be very useful to understand a little about what tests your doctor can order, what their limitations are, and what you can do with the information.

ELECTROCARDIOGRAM (ECG OR EKG)

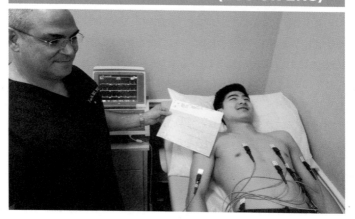

What is it? The ECG is a quick, simple test that tells us what rhythm your heart is in at that moment, and it infers your heart's structure and function. ECGs can change in an instant, so it is a test often repeated.

What are its limits? It only infers your heart's structure and function, and only as it is *in that moment.* You can have a "normal" ECG and still have major heart issues. It is NOT a complete test of your heart's health.

When do I want one? In adulthood at baseline, regularly with physicals, and any time there may be a relevant change.

What does it tell me? An ECG is like a vital sign (such as your blood pressure). It is a basic piece of information about your health that can change at any time, even minute-to-minute.

ECHOCARDIOGRAM (ECHO)

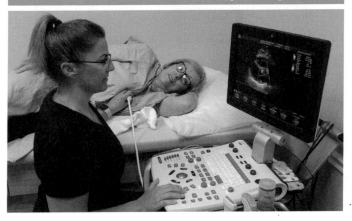

What is it? The echo is an ultrasound of your heart. It will tell you exactly what your heart's structure and function is. It will tell you the strength of your heart, whether it has been damaged, how it works, how well your blood pressure has been controlled. It also gives a lot of information about your risk of AFib and your stroke risk in general.

What are its limits? By itself, it only shows how your heart is working when you are at rest. It needs to be combined with an exercise test to know how well your heart works under stress.

When do I want one? When you have the first concern for high blood pressure; when you have any symptoms at all (breathlessness, chest discomfort, dizziness, irregular heartbeats, fatigue... anything); or if your ECG has any changes or abnormalities. You do not need to see a cardiologist to have an echo, but it helps to understand what to do with the information it is giving you.

What does it tell me? Everything. The echo tells your doctor if you need medicine for blood pressure, if you need different medicine, if you need something to improve your heart's health, and if you need to be concerned about AFib. An echo is essentially an advanced physical exam of your heart, and it may be repeated to track your heart's health.

STRESS TEST/STRESS ECHOCARDIOGRAM

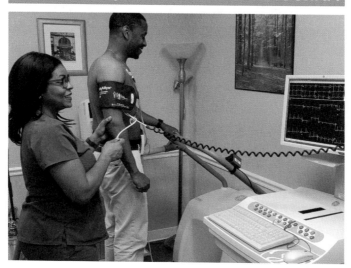

What is it? Getting on a treadmill to see how you respond to physical activity and getting pictures of your heart with ultrasound.

What are its limits? To do this test, you must have a skilled technician, and you need to be able to walk (at least a little). Note: A stress test without imaging (like an echo or the nuclear imaging described on the next page) is of very little value. It will confirm your ability to exercise, but little more. A stress test MUST include imaging to provide useful information about your heart's health and safety. Simple exercise testing can be done by a technologist, but a stress echo requires a cardiologist as well as a technician. In general, primary care physicians do not have the training or equipment to do this.

When do I want one? As soon as you are at risk for heart and vascular disease. For example, anyone with diabetes should have this done by age 50. Just about everyone is at risk for vascular disease by age 65.

What does it tell me? Everything. A stress echo is like taking a car for a test drive and watching the engine running at full speed. If everything works, you know you have a good engine, and if something doesn't work, you can see what it is. It will tell you your risk of heart attack. It will tell you the limits of your ability to exercise. It will guide therapy for the prevention of heart attacks and heart failure—which medications are likely to be useful and why. It identifies high- and low-risk situations, and it indicates whether you should have more invasive treatments.

NUCLEAR STRESS TEST

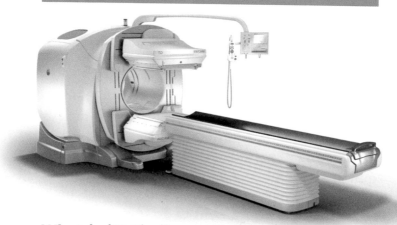

What is it? Similar to a stress echo, nuclear stress testing involves taking pictures of the heart both before and after some form of stress. The pictures are obtained by injecting radioactive material that collects in the heart and can be seen with special cameras. It is an excellent test to determine how well blood flows to the heart, since the radioactive material can only reach the heart if the blood flow is not blocked. There is more than one way to create stress. A standard treadmill can be used, or you can be injected with a medication that simulates stress. This is especially helpful for people who cannot walk.

What are its limits? If a medication (or chemical) stress test is done, it will not tell you anything about your functional capacity or symptoms. It does not demonstrate your heart's function nearly as well as an echo. Also, there is a considerable amount of radiation, especially if you need to repeat the test regularly.

When do I want one? It is a common form of stress test as an alternative to a stress echo. It is used for all of the same reasons as a stress echo. It does not require the same level of technical expertise, so it is easier to perform.

What does it tell me? A nuclear stress test can guide medical therapy or indicate whether you might benefit from more invasive procedures.

CARDIAC CT (CAT SCAN)/CT ANGIOGRAM

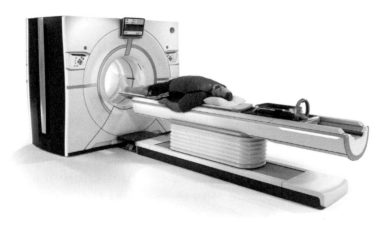

What is it? A CT scan involves an injection of dye and X-rays to create a picture of the arteries to the heart. It can tell you if your arteries are beginning to age (by measuring degree of calcification or hardening). It can indicate whether there is blockage in the arteries to the heart.

What are its limits? It does not tell you about your heart's function. It does not always correlate with risk. Most people have some degree of abnormality, so it tends to prompt additional testing (such as a stress test). It requires considerable dye and radiation, and serial testing may not correlate with progression of disease or help guide therapy.

When do I want one? It is often used as a tool to prompt people to see a cardiologist, or to prompt them to start taking medications if they are otherwise reluctant. It can be very useful in some people with established disease.

What does it tell me? Not much. If perfectly normal, it can reassure you that you are not at high risk. One of the most important things you can do with an abnormal CT scan is to see a cardiologist for a stress test (stress echo or nuclear stress test). Then again, you don't have to have a CT scan to see a cardiologist or get a stress test. It is helpful as a confirmatory test when stress test results are unclear.

HOLTER MONITOR

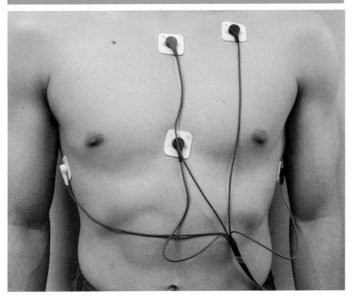

What is it? A Holter monitor is a small device that records your heart's ECG for 24–48 hours.

What are its limits? The Holter monitor will only record what your heart is doing for the day you are wearing it. Infrequent events, such as intermittent AFib, may not happen on the day you are wearing it.

When do I want one? When it is helpful to know the health of your heart's conduction system (aka, your natural pacemaker). If you have symptoms of AFib, or you are at risk of AFib. It is often not enough information, but it is a very good and easy place to start.

NAVIGATING (WITH) YOUR DOCTOR

What does it tell me? If you're lucky, you may catch AFib or an arrhythmia. It can also guide medical therapy and direct which medications may be helpful for you. It can identify people at higher risk for AFib and thus define who might benefit from further monitoring.

WEARABLE CARDIAC MONITORS

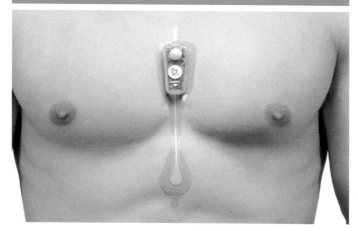

What is it? There are many variations of monitors that allow for monitoring the heart for a longer period of time, typically two to four weeks. They have the advantage over a Holter monitor in that they record data for a longer period of time.

What are its limits? In practical terms, they require some form of adhesive to the skin, which can be challenging to tolerate for more than about a week. Also, even four weeks may not be enough time to catch an infrequent event.

When do I want one? If you are concerned that you may be having AFib (or any irregular heartbeat), and you do not want a long-term monitor (see "Implantable Cardiac Monitors").

What does it tell me? If you capture an episode of AFib, then it guides how you can prevent strokes.

EVENT/COMMERCIAL CARDIAC MONITORS

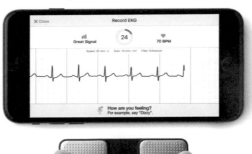

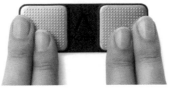

What is it? These monitors are commercial devices that can turn your cell phone into a portable ECG machine to allow you to record your heart's rhythm and potentially email it to your doctor.

What are its limits? It will only work when you activate it. If events happen quickly, or if you have asymptomatic AFib, you may miss recording it.

When do I want one? If you have symptoms, specifically irregular heartbeats or palpitations, that are too infrequent to catch with a wearable monitor, and you are relatively facile with your cell phone.

What does it tell me? If you capture an episode of AFib, then it can help guide how you can prevent strokes.

IMPLANTABLE CARDIAC MONITORS
(Implantable Loop Recorders)

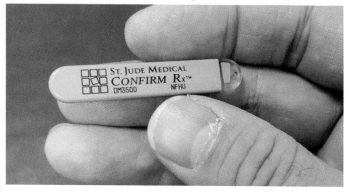

What is it? This type of monitor is a microchip that is injected under the skin. It records your ECG continuously 24 hours a day and will automatically alert your doctor if you have AFib or any irregular heartbeat. It also allows you to send ECGs to your doctor anytime you have symptoms. It is always on, and it has a complete memory. Nothing is ever missed. The battery lasts for two to three years.

What are its limits? You need to get one stitch.

When do I want one? When you are worried you may have AFib and can no longer wear a monitor taped to your chest. When you have palpitations or unexplained symptoms.

What does it tell me? Everything. The information is complete. It removes all doubt and mystery as to what your heart is doing. It is therefore a very effective way to guide therapy, especially for AFib.

CAROTID/VASCULAR ULTRASOUND

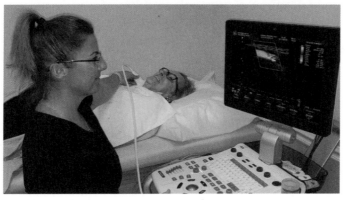

What is it? An ultrasound allows you to see into and through the wall of the arteries to determine your arterial health.

What are its limits? When done by non-cardiovascular doctors, or as a health fair screening tool, the test may be imprecise or vague. You want a high-resolution study.

When do I want one? As soon as you are old enough to be concerned about your vascular aging. Like stress testing, it depends on your risk profile, but the baseline is age 50 (especially if you have any risk factors). Follow up periodically to evaluate for disease progression.

What does it tell me? This test is one of the most useful tests in guiding medical therapy. It shows progression of disease and characterizes risk. It can tell you when to start medical therapy, and when to increase or change medical therapy. There are now many new medical options to prevent plaque progression and lower stroke risk.

IN SUMMARY, THE GUIDELINES FOR CARDIOVASCULAR TESTING ARE:

Who: Everyone

When: Ten years younger than the age of the youngest relative who has heart or vascular disease, at age 40–50 (depending on risk) for some baseline information, and after age 65.

What: Start with your internist/primary care doctor. Analyze your risk. Get an echo. Have a stress test when it's time. Know that your stress test must have some form of imaging with it to be useful. Look at your carotid arteries. Get a monitor of some sort when concerned about AFib.

Why: It matters. It changes what you can do to prevent strokes.

NOTES:

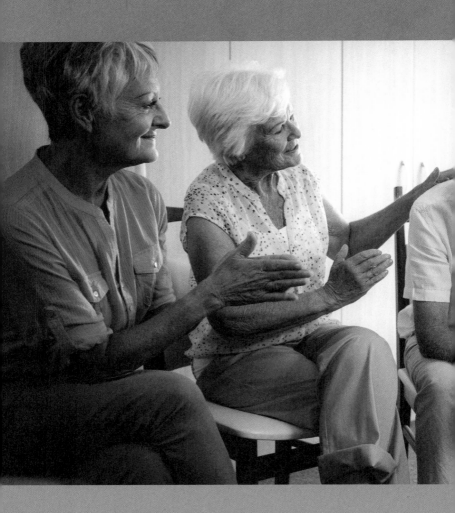

CHAPTER 8

CONSIDERING OTHERS

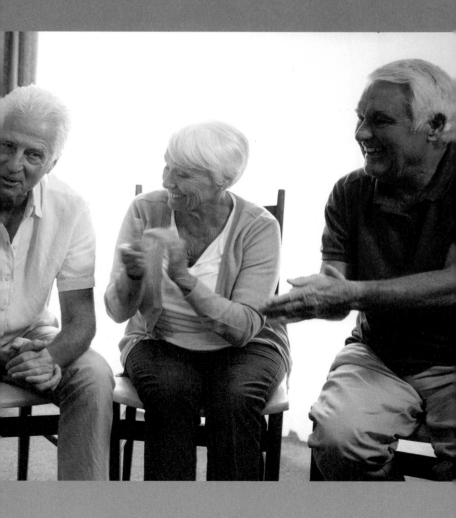

When I was in kindergarten, we were all supposed to tell our class what our fathers did for a living. My father worked for the Department of Health, Education and Welfare (now HHS). So, naturally, I hadn't the faintest idea what he did.

So, I went home and asked. His answer started, "Son, first we need to define the word *health*."

To this day, I'm not sure I know what he did. But his initial response was valid. What exactly is health? When I train medical students, I like to emphasize to them that everything we do should be for one of two reasons: to help someone live longer or to help them feel better. We should always be clear on why we are doing something.

Sometimes we do one at the expense of the other. There are a great many things we can do to make us feel good, but they may shorten our lives. Likewise, sometimes doctors will ask us to do things to lengthen our lives that may not be very pleasant.

When we are doing something for our health, we should ask if it will make us live longer or feel better.

We very commonly associate fitness with health. We look at athletes and marvel at what they do, and we think, wow, they're healthy. And then you hear about someone dying unexpectedly. Fitness is what our body can do and how well it can do it. Health is more than that. It also includes whether we are likely to die or suffer damage. Health asks, are we going to live as long as we want, and are we going to feel as well as we want?

Health and fitness are not the same thing.
This works both ways. I have a patient who is lean and fit as can be. He runs marathons. He never felt bad or complained a day in his life. He never took a pill. But he had a massive buildup of plaque. He collapsed without warning, survived, had bypass surgery, and now (at age 85) has a pacemaker and is back to running marathons. He has always been fit, but he has not always been healthy.

Fitness alone does not guarantee health. Medicines are often necessary.
I also have a patient who weighs so much that I could not put him on my treadmill (which will not support someone over 450 pounds). He could not walk across the waiting room without becoming breathless. He takes a dozen medications at least. Since I could barely see or test his heart, I had him undergo a heart catheterization (an invasive test to see if he had any plaque in his coronary arteries). His arteries were as clean as a whistle, and his cardiac function was perfectly normal. He took all the

pills that we asked him to, so we prevented any damage to his heart. He actually had a healthy heart, but he was not at all fit.

There is no pill for fitness.
Neither of these two patients had an ideal life. One nearly died from asymptomatic plaque buildup because he didn't think he needed to see a doctor or take a pill. One takes all the pills he needs to and has a perfectly working heart but thought it was not necessary to stay fit.

What do these two men have in common? They each had a firm belief in how they wanted to manage their lives. That, of course, is a polite way of saying they were somewhat stubborn.

Would you rather be fit and drop dead early, or unfit and live miserably? How about neither?

Your doctor can give you pills, but you have to keep yourself fit.
Exercise sounds too much like an event. Fitness is a lifestyle. It should be like brushing your teeth. It's not an event, but part of your daily routine.

Likely, everything you've ever heard about exercise is true, but let me give you the cardiovascular short course. There are three basic types of exercise: cardiovascular (aerobic), strength training (anaerobic), and balance/ coordination/flexibility exercises. They are all good and all important. A balanced exercise program will include variable elements of all three. But your heart actually doesn't care if you can pick up a bus or bend over backward and touch your head to the floor. Your heart and circulation really want regular cardiovascular exercise.

Our hearts would rather we be marathon runners than sprinters or power-lifters.
What's more, our hearts don't need us to run at all. Running hurts my knees (and back and ankles and hips and feet). Walking is actually quite good. If you do nothing else, walk every day.

But there's another point to consider: Don't go too hard. We have a tendency to try to work out really hard, get very tired, and then quit. That will not help you. Everyone asks me, how hard they should work out, but this is the wrong question. The right question is how often. The answer: every day. The next right question is for how long. The answer: 30–60 minutes.

When exercising, think frequency first. Duration second. Intensity last.
How much you do and how regularly you do it is much more important in the beginning than how hard. You must create the habit of fitness. Once you have a routine, then you can work on customizing it to what works for your body and

CONSIDERING OTHERS

your life. Start the habit first. I also am often asked, "What type of exercise monitor should I get?" The answer: A wall calendar. Mark off a box every day to track that you did something. Then get a watch to see if you were moving for at least 30 minutes. Then go faster.

Just as exercise does not guarantee our health, neither does diet.
Currently, if you search "diet books for health" on Amazon, you will find over 100,000 titles. This is not one of them. Remember, heart disease is not a singular thing. A healthy brain requires a healthy heart. There is not a direct path between food and heart damage or brain damage.

Food is not directly toxic to the heart or brain.
That being said, nutrition matters. Nutrition, like fitness, should be a way of life, not just a one-time diet. The arc from diet to heart disease goes through metabolism and accelerated vascular aging. That means we need to avoid diabetes.

If we consume calories faster than we burn them off, we end up storing them. We then build up fat and can become obese. The formula is: Calories eaten minus calories burned equals calories kept (or lost). If we don't burn off what we eat, then we gain weight. Obesity leads to diabetes. When that happens, the sugar levels in our blood get higher, and we become resistant to insulin (which helps us metabolize sugar).

Obesity leads to diabetes, which accelerates vascular aging and increases the workload on the heart.
Our genetics have largely programmed us to store calories more readily as we get older. It used to take a lot of energy to get food. We had to burn calories to get calories. We now live in a world where we have nearly infinite calories at our fingertips with no physical effort. (I can use my cell phone and people will bring me calories. I only have to get up to answer the door.) Our balance between calories burned and calories consumed has skewed.

One hundred thousand years ago, humans expended a lot of energy in order to get food. Hunting a woolly mammoth was hard work. Today, calories are too easy to come by, and we are prone to obesity and diabetes. Today, more people die of vascular disease than starvation.

For better or worse, our metabolic rate usually declines with age. That means for the same diet and the same activity level, you will start to gain weight. If you want to keep eating the same food, you're going to have to increase your exercise, or you'll gain weight.

What can we do? All diets have one thing in common: calorie reduction.

How much we eat always matters. What we eat is a more complex question.

Genetics matter. The Mediterranean diet has been shown in several studies to decrease the likelihood of diabetes and thus reduce the risk of heart disease. That's great, but did you check to see where those studies were done? The latest one (published in the *New England Journal of Medicine* no less), was done entirely in Spain. It also works in Italy, Greece, and Lebanon.

So, if you are genetically Mediterranean, eat like your grandparents did.

Come to think of it, that is generally good advice. In Washington, DC, we commonly see international visitors. A lot of them have never been to this country before and have never experienced the wonders of American food. (They serve an awesome Half-Smoke at Nationals Ballpark.) After a year of this dietary change, many of our visitors will have severe weight gain and diabetes.

When considering diet, you must consider your genetics. You may need to eat like your grandparents did (in order to have a diet that you can metabolize).

Americans are largely descended from immigrants. We have the most genetic diversity on the planet, and we have an awesome array of culinary possibilities. Don't eat too much, and check with your doctor to make sure you are not developing diabetes.

So, the first part of this chapter includes the things you need to do for yourself—namely, stay fit and have good nutrition. Now comes Part 2: working with your doctor. I will assume that you are motivated to be healthy. But perhaps you also have a stubborn streak.

It's just as wrong to think that we can do everything for ourselves as it is to think that our doctors can do everything for us.
Stubbornness of all sorts can get us killed, or worse. It can lead to unnecessary strokes, brain damage, and vascular dementia.

So, a note on how we make decisions: Remember the old *Star Trek* series from the '60s? I always related to Spock. He was the dispassionate science officer who made decisions based on logic and reason. His counterpart was Dr. McCoy, who seemed to be driven by passion and emotion. When it comes to health, I would like to think that we are all driven by reasoned thought, but in truth, to some degree or another, we can be driven by emotions. In other words, my friend "Dr. Feel Good" had a point. What we believe is often driven by how we feel as much as what we think.

I would tend to encourage people to make decisions through reason, but I have often found that our preconceived beliefs and emotions often drive decision making that can lead to less than optimal outcomes. That is my polite way of saying that people often make poor choices.

When making choices about your health care, it is usually helpful to balance emotion with thought. Think through your decisions. One of the troubles with poor choices is that we can damage our brains. We can have strokes. We can encourage vascular dementia. When that happens, the person who has lost brain function is not the only one who suffers. Disability and loss of brain function is the path to loss of independence. It creates a burden on everyone else.

So, if you know someone, perhaps a parent or a spouse or some family member whom you care about, and you don't think they are making the best personal choices in protecting their health (and protecting their brains!), then the best we can do is try to offer them other, better choices.

Here are some of the most common challenges I see. I call this "THE LITANY OF STUBBORNNESS."

"I don't need to see a doctor. I'm healthy."
Remember, health and fitness are not the same thing. The body can be a lot like a car. You wouldn't buy a car just because it looks good on the outside. You want to make sure the motor is not about to break down. You only know how well the motor works if you check it out. Cars require maintenance. Moving parts wear out. You don't want to go looking for a mechanic after your engine has caught fire. It is always best to have a relationship with a doctor before you have a problem.
Health and fitness are not the same thing.

"I don't trust doctors."
Good for you. Neither do I. They can, however, be useful. Ask your doctor to explain to you why they are recommending what they are. Remember, everything we do in medicine should serve to help us either live longer or feel better. Ask your doctor what the goals are. Make sure you and your doctor share the same goals.
Doctors really do want to help.

CONSIDERING OTHERS

"My mother was fine until she went to see a doctor, and then she died."

Looking fine and being healthy are not the same thing. If she waited until she felt bad about something, in all likelihood, she missed chances to have prevented whatever it was that killed her (especially if it was heart and vascular disease).

Denial and avoidance are deadly.

"But I'm thin."

Uggh. Being thin means you are thin. It doesn't mean that you are genetically exempt from disease or aging. If you are thin because you are fit and exercise a lot, that's great—but smokers are some of the thinnest people around, and they are not exactly healthy.

How you look on the inside and how you look on the outside are not the same.

"I only eat _____." (Fill in the blank: vegetables, low fat, non-processed, whole-grain imported paleo seeds from a mountain in Tibet.) "My cholesterol is fine."

We don't treat cholesterol for the sake of the number. We promote vascular health and prevent strokes. The best diet in the world does not change genetics or take away the effects of time.

Doctors treat people, not numbers.

"I'm healthy. I don't want to take pills."
Think of them as vitamins for your blood vessels. What do you have to lose? They're almost all generic and cheap.
We live in the 21st century. The miracles of modern medicine only work if we take the pills.

"I heard that statins are awful. They cause joint and muscle pain."
In all major studies, about 5% of people who take statins report aches and pains. In the same studies, 5% of people on a placebo (a sugar pill) will also report aches and pains. When you do a blinded crossover (where subjects switch back and forth between a pill and a placebo), on average, no one can tell if they are on a statin or not.

What that means, really, is that 5% of us readily get aches and pains. Personally, I had many aches and pains before I started my statin. It is possible that someone can feel worse on a particular statin, but fortunately, there are many to choose from, and they are not the same (especially in terms of side effects).

If your doctor recommends a statin (and they eventually will), you should try it. If you think you are prone to aches and pains, you will have aches and pains after you

CONSIDERING OTHERS

start the statin as well. You can work with your doctor. You can switch statins. You can add the dietary supplement coenzyme Q10, which in some people eliminates the aches and pains. You can take microdoses of statins. You can try taking it once a week. There is a lot you can do, but it helps to have a relationship with your doctor for guidance. Remember, the goal is prevention of brain damage, and statins are very good at doing that. Finding something you can take is worth the effort.

Statins really are a miracle of modern medicine. When it's time, give them a try.

"I heard that statins cause dementia."

This is essentially an internet-driven hoax. Statins are extraordinarily valuable. They prevent strokes. They prevent brain damage. They also prevent heart attacks and premature death. There is a reason people are living longer today than they were a generation ago. Remember, the Social Security age was set at 65 because life expectancy at the time was only 63. Give a lot of credit to statins.

Just because you heard something at a party or on the internet doesn't make it true.

"I don't want to take a baby aspirin because I bruise."

(You know who you are, Mom.) Bruising is a nuisance. But clotting kills. If you clot something off, you kill it. We all typically die when we clot off the heart or brain. We can live with the bruises.

Strokes and heart attacks are caused by clots. Prevent them.

"I don't want to take a blood thinner because I might bleed."

Well, especially if you have AFib, don't tell me what you don't want to do. Tell me what you are going to do. What is your risk of a stroke if you choose to do nothing? Do you really want to saddle your family with that risk? Yes, people can bleed, but that is largely treatable. Yes, there is a very small chance of death from bleeding, but there is a large chance of disability and brain damage when you clot. If you are going to choose to do nothing, make sure you really, really know what that means for you and for the people who have to take care of you.

We always balance the risk of bleeding versus the risk of clotting.

CONSIDERING OTHERS

"I don't want to take these new blood thinners (like Xarelto and Eliquis). My doctor says you can't reverse them. What if I'm in an accident?"

First of all, your doctor is wrong and outdated. Second, the best way to treat bleeding is to not bleed at all, and the 21st-century stroke prevention agents produce a lot less bleeding than the old-fashioned rat poison that you may have been taking. Third, if you are in an accident, you don't treat bleeding by feeding people vegetables. (What? Yes, that is fundamentally how you "reverse" warfarin. It takes about a day.)

Modern blood thinners are safer and more effective than older alternatives.

"I don't feel anything. Why do I have to take a pill to prevent strokes?

Most AFib is asymptomatic. So is plaque for that matter. If your doctor is recommending a pill to prevent strokes, it's for a reason. Just ask what the reason is. Just because you don't have symptoms doesn't mean you won't benefit from medications.

Symptoms do not predict risk.

"Why do I need a heart monitor? Why do I need any of these tests?"

Because heart disease is a silent killer.

But it is not invisible. We can see it, but we have to look. It's not hard.

You only know your health if you look.

"I've always had a slow heartbeat. I've always been healthy."

Yes, but you've never been 75 years old before. Your heart is going to get slower with age. Do you really think that your body hasn't changed in the last 50 years? When your heart is slow, you are simply not pumping as much blood. At some point, that will become a problem. It will affect your brain.

This phenomenon, in fact, is one of the hardest to deal with. If your brain is slowly affected by a chronically slow heart, you are usually not aware of it. Other people will just see you fade away.

Pacemakers are a reward for healthy people who live long enough to benefit from them.

Ultimately, doctors are just here to give you their best advice. The final choices are always up to you. Another of my favorite patients (a true scholar) once told me that there was once an implicit pact between doctors and patients. Doctors always had their patient's best interest at heart. They used their extensive training,

CONSIDERING OTHERS

experience, and personal knowledge of their patient to give their best advice, which used to be called "doctor's orders." And people followed their doctor's orders.

Today, we live in the information age. Technology abounds. Expectations have changed. Everyone is unique, and "Endowed by their Creator to certain unalienable rights, that among these are Life, Liberty and the Pursuit of Happiness."

Well, doctors can give you advice about how to prolong life. You have the liberty to take the advice or not. And ultimately, how you pursue happiness is up to you. We're just here to help.

NOTES:

THE "AFTER PART":
ANSWERS AT THE END OF THE BOOK

My daughter, who, like her mother, is smarter than I am, informed me that the best movies have an "after part" at the end of the credits. She also has discovered that the best school-books have answers in the back. So, here are the answers (in short form).

To keep your brain (and yourself as a whole) healthy, know the answers to the questions:

1. What is the health of my heart and circulation?
2. What can I do, or what can I do differently to keep my circulation working as SAFELY and EFFICIENTLY as possible?

To prevent strokes and vascular dementia:

1. Establish a relationship with a physician.
2. Know the health of your heart.
3. Know the health of your arteries
4. Know the regularity of your heartbeat.
5. Know if it's time to take a medicine to prevent plaque buildup in your arteries and or to prevent a blood clot.

The best way to treat a stroke is to not have one in the first place.

These are the key takeaways you should remember:

- Plaque in blood vessels, or atherosclerosis, is not a disease. It is a natural part of aging.

- Statin medications directly prevent vascular inflammation and plaque growth. They are vascular protective medications, not just cholesterol medications.

- There is (almost) no such thing as heart disease. It's mostly just natural aging.

- You are not immune from aging.

- Aging is predictable, measurable, and manageable.

- Atrial fibrillation, or AFib, is very common, and it is a major reason why we have strokes.

- Atrial fibrillation is often asymptomatic, but it still puts you at risk for a stroke whether you feel it or not.

- Atrial fibrillation is part of the aging process. It may be inevitable if we live long enough.

- You don't cure AFib. You MANAGE it.

- If you want to know if you are having AFib, you have to monitor for it.

- When you have any AFib at all, you must ask, what am I doing to prevent strokes?

YOU CAN PREVENT A STROKE

- If you have AFib, you should be on a stroke prevention medication like Xarelto or Eliquis, or have a good reason why you are not.

- Healthy brains require healthy hearts. You must maintain good blood flow to the brain.

- Blood flow matters more than blood pressure.

- Our blood flow depends heavily (but not exclusively) on our heart rate.

- If you have too slow a heart rate, or too many pauses without a heartbeat, you will damage your brain from lack of blood flow.

- The problems from a slow heart can be prevented with a pacemaker.

- Heart and vascular disease is a silent killer, but it is not invisible. We can see it.

- If you want to know how healthy something is, look at it.

- Trust, but verify. If you want to know your heart's function, test it.

- The health of your heart and circulation is a knowable thing. But you have to ask the questions.

- When we are doing something for our health, we should ask whether it is going to make us live longer or feel better.

- Health and fitness are not the same thing.

These are the major points of this book. To understand them in context, please read, or re-read, the earlier chapters. Share this book with friends. Better yet, have them buy one themselves.

I do tell all of my patients that I want them to follow up with my daughter, who I hope will take over my practice. But, as she is only in middle school, they're going to have to wait quite a while. If we work together and they follow the guidance in this book, I expect them to get there, without having a stroke along the way.

PHOTO CREDITS

"Late Complications of Atherosclerosis."
https://commons.wikimedia.org/wiki/File:Late_
complications_of_atherosclerosis.PNG

"Carotid Artery Diagram."
https://commons.wikimedia.org/wikiFile:Blau-
sen_0170_CarotidArteries.png) Blausen.com.staff
(2014).

"Medical gallery of Blausen Medical 2014".
WikiJournal of Medicine 1 (2). DOI:10.15347/
wjm/2014.010. ISSN 2002-4436.

"Heart Rate Target Chart."
http://www.briody-fitnessnhealth.com/targetheart-
rate.html

"Diagram of the Human Heart."
https://en.wikipedia.org/wiki/File:Diagram_of_
the_human_heart_(cropped).svg
Author: Eric Pierce, 2006.

**"The United States Marine Corps Band
(The President's Own) marches down 15th Street
during the 1997 presidential inaugural parade."**
https://commons.wikimedia.org/wiki/
File:President%27s_Own_during_1997_Inaugural_
parade.JPEG
Author: Duncan Graham, 1997.

"Atrial Fibrillation (AF)" and **"Normal Sinus Rhythm
(NSR)"**
Copyright 2016 by Jason Winter. Reprinted by
permission.

ACKNOWLEDGMENTS

We are enormously grateful to the many people who helped with this project – not only the book, but with the foundation as a whole. A complete list would be too long to print, but we would like to thank a few special people. First, several folk were essential in supporting the foundation, including Jim Lemon (go Senators!), Carol and Henry Goldberg, Terry Eakin, and Paul and Marilynn Yentis.

We are also grateful to the team at Rosetta Books who took on the project and made the words look so good, especially Arthur Klebanoff, Brian Skulnik, and Michelle Weyenberg.

Thanks to our staff (who often doubled as models), including Frank Pita, Cozette Powell, Denise Hitt, Tony Pruitt, Sam Han, Angela (the boss) Jones, and Maria, Daja and Lekeisha (who had enough sense to stay out of pictures), as well as the Steves (Houck and and Tabb) who do real work; and our early reviewers, Hugh Caulkins, Ed Kasper, Zayd Eldadah, Mike Dennin (get his book, it's really good!), and Mike Hildreth.

And most of all, we are grateful to Bill Lilley, the Midwife of this entire project, without whose guidance and help, this would never have happened.